Comprehensive Care for Complex Patients

The Medical–Psychiatric Coordinating Physician Model

Comprehensive Care for Complex Patients

The Medical–Psychiatric Coordinating Physician Model

Steven A. Frankel, MD

Clinical Associate Professor, University of California School of Medicine, San Francisco, and Director, Center for Collaborative Psychiatry, Psychology, and Medicine, Kentfield, CA, USA

James A. Bourgeois, OD, MD

Professor, Department of Psychiatry & Behavioural Neurosciences, Michael G. DeGroote School of Medicine, Faculty of Health Sciences, McMaster University, Ontario, Canada

Philip Erdberg, PhD

Assistant Clinical Professor, University of California School of Medicine, San Francisco, CA, USA

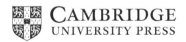

CAMBRIDGE
UNIVERSITY PRESS

CAMBRIDGE UNIVERSITY PRESS
Cambridge, New York, Melbourne, Madrid, Cape Town,
Singapore, São Paulo, Delhi, Mexico City

Cambridge University Press
The Edinburgh Building, Cambridge CB2 8RU, UK

Published in the United States of America by
Cambridge University Press, New York

www.cambridge.org
Information on this title: www.cambridge.org/9781107025158

First published 2013

Printed and bound in the United Kingdom by the MPG Books Group

A catalogue record for this publication is available from the British Library

Library of Congress Cataloging-in-Publication Data

Frankel, Steven A.
    Comprehensive care for complex patients : the medical-psychiatric coordinating physician model /
Steven A. Frankel, James A. Bourgeois, Philip Erdberg.
        p.   cm.
    Includes bibliographical references and index.
    ISBN 978-1-107-02515-8 (Hardback)
    1. Psychiatry.   2. Patients–Mental health.   3. Psychotherapy.   4. Physician and patient.
I. Bourgeois, James.   II. Erdberg, Philip.   III. Title.
    RC454.4.F72 2013
    616.89–dc23

                                                                            2012017178

ISBN 978-1-107-02515-8 Hardback

Contents

Forewords, James Rundell MD, Roger Kathol MD, and
Wolfgang Söllner, MD   *page* vii
Preface   xi
Endorsements   xiii
Acknowledgments   xviii

Section 1 Introduction

1   Complex treatments: the evolving place for a medical–psychiatric
    coordinating physician   1

Section 2 Guidance for negotiating clinical complexity

2   Beyond the physician–patient model: the value of a treatment
    team for dealing with clinical complexity   25

3   Sorting out clinical complexity: medical and psychometric
    testing   36

4   The limitations of algorithms: details of two "clinically
    complex" treatments   48

5   Negotiating the subjectivity and inter-subjectivity of the
    clinical field: the complexity inherent in clinical work   65

Section 3 Clinical decisions and their execution: accuracy within complexity

6   The intersection of data and clinical judgment: the place of
    subjectivity in treatment decisions   81

7   Clinical strategy: grappling with treatment complexity   91

8   Working consensus: the importance of physician–patient
     collaboration   105

9   Linking truing measures: technical and interpersonal precision
     in work with complex cases   119

Section 4 The application of the model: the medical–psychiatric coordinating physician

10   Managing complex treatments: the medical–psychiatric
     coordinating physician   133

11   The medical–psychiatric coordinating physician: clinical
     role, training models, costs, and future directions   148

     References   169
     Index   178

Forewords

There is increasing emphasis on integration of mental health and medical services. Integrated behavioral health models are emerging with compelling evidence for clinical and cost effectiveness. Experts in these models have found that patients in these integrated programs who have highly complex co-morbid psychiatric and medical conditions require additional attention to ensure optimal outcomes.

The authors of this timely text long ago developed a model, through years of clinical experience, to manage these most complex patients. Their proposition is refreshing just in time for an era in which emerging models of accountable care will require novel solutions that engage, embrace, and actively manage complex patients instead of avoiding them and deferring or spinning off their care.

For patients requiring a higher degree of intervention than psychiatric advice, psychiatric consultation, and nurse or social work case management, the notion of the seasoned psychiatrist being the air traffic controller for the patient's overall care, in addition to serving as the treating psychiatrist, is proposed. The authors have studied their outcomes and present them in the text. They provide numerous illustrative case examples of how their psychiatrist-led team approach works with real patients. They describe how the medical psychiatric coordinating physician operates in simultaneous macroscopic and microscopic roles. Their model is compelling; this text is a must-read.

James Rundell, MD
Vice-Chair, Psychiatry and Psychology, Mayo clinic, USA

From my perspective, perhaps the greatest contribution of this book by Frankel, Bourgeois, and Erdberg is its coverage of the "complexity" approach to care. Few physicians, let alone psychiatrists, have an appreciation of the connection between chronic complicated illnesses and non-illness related factors that lead to treatment resistance, persistent illness, high health costs, and personal and functional impairment. This book serves as a primer for psychiatrists interested in addressing the needs of complicated patients at the interface of medicine and psychiatry on complexity theory and the application of assessment techniques that allow medical psychiatric coordinating physicians (MPCPs) or health professionals, such as care/case managers under their supervision, to connect clinical and non-clinical complexity needs through coordinated service delivery.

I have known Drs. Frankel and Bourgeois for several years, since we all have an interest in improving the care of primary and specialty medical patients with psychiatric co-morbidity. Both are quality physicians and innovative thinkers. Our common interest has led to a number of stimulating discussions about clinical approaches that can be considered for use when health and life complexity overtax standard care capabilities and thus require innovative approaches to reverse persistent health, life, and cost problems. Dr. Frankel has used one such approach for a number of years, i.e., a psychiatrist-centric model in which MPCPs take on the role of physical and mental health team lead for patients with significant psychiatric contributions to their health outcomes. It is this model and the patient cases exposed to it that forms the unique content of this book.

The complexity, rather than a disease, approach to patients described in the book draws on the experience and expertise of a group of researchers in Europe. The INTERMED group has been instrumental in supplying a methodology to health system professionals that allows them to identify patients at high risk for poor outcomes using a multi-domain (biopsychosocial and health system) assessment system. Results of the complexity assessment inform the direction of care delivery needed to reverse poor clinical and cost outcomes. Understanding this concept alone makes this book a valuable read.

Psychiatrists with training in psychosomatic medicine (consultation-liaison (CL) psychiatrists) or those who have completed joint residencies (internal medicine and psychiatry; family practice and psychiatry; psychiatry, child psychiatry, and pediatrics) are an ideal group to take ownership of patients with health complexity, since they have interest and expertise that allows them to take on the role of MPCPs described in the book. While these would be a group for which the book would provide an informative read, general psychiatrists would also benefit, since their roles in the future will include greater clinical activity and a better understanding of psychiatric care in the primary and specialty medical sector. Furthermore, there are far too few CL or jointly trained psychiatrists to assume accountability for medical/surgical patients with complex health needs.

This leads to a discussion of what I consider a major concern associated with use of the MPCP model *per se* as described in the book. The model defines an approach to complex patients with the MPCP at the center of activity, i.e., the coordinator of all care (medical and psychiatric). While this has clear advantages in terms of having a highly qualified practitioner in change, Drs. Frankel and Bourgeois and I have had several debates on just how practical the MPCP approach is, given the short supply of psychiatrists willing to practice in the medical sector, let alone the number of CL or jointly trained physicians. This, along with other factors, could hamper safe, effective, outcome changing, and sustainable implementation, such as: (1) which patients should be targeted for assignment to a MPCP; (2) how the MPCP will interact with primary and specialty care physicians and share responsibility for physical illness decision-making; (3) who will be included among the coordinated care teams and how they will communicate when not part of a closed system; (4) how many complex patients can be assigned to a MPCP before workload exhausts capacity to create outcome change; and (5) who will pay for the MPCP services delivered at a rate that covers professional costs.

In a sense, the fact that these questions loom is good. Readers will be stimulated to come up with either answers or alternatives to the approach described in the book. Patients with health complexity are clearly a group that requires additional thought by innovative clinicians and health system administrators, since they constitute the small percentage of patients (2% to 10%) that use 30% to 70% of health resources, largely due to poorly treated and thus persistent clinical disorders. New ways to address the health needs of these patients are required. The MPCP model provides one concrete suggestion on how better outcomes for these patients might be addressed. It also stimulates thought about alternatives.

My discussions with Drs. Frankel and Bourgeois have certainly motivated me to think more concretely about substitutes or model offshoots that might be considered as more practical choices for management of complex patients. For instance, there is good data now showing that care managers are effective in reversing complex patient outcomes when supervised by clinicians with the expertise to consider alternative or escalated care when improvement is not occurring. Would routine use of care managers be a logical extension of the MPCP model, allowing expansion of reach for the MPCP to a larger population of patients? These and many other options should be considered as readers peruse this psychiatrist-centric model.

Roger Kathol. MD
Professor of Internal Medicine and Psychiatry, University of Minnesota, USA

Despite the existence of several theoretical and practical approaches for overcoming the mind-body divide, modern medicine is still characterized by fragmented care, particularly for more difficult cases such as those involving chronic and complex illness. These patients typically find themselves deprived of sorely needed comprehensive and personalized care.

With this book, the authors present a new model confronting the challenges of providing care for complex patients with psychiatric comorbidity. It features a physician with a new role, that of the Medical–Psychiatric Coordinating Physician (MPCP). Besides his or her traditional 'microscopic', specialization i.e. clinical tasks within his or her specialty (psychiatry, internal medicine or family medicine), that physician assumes the 'macroscopic' tasks of actively enhancing interdisciplinary collaboration and leading a multi-professional team. By taking on these roles, that physician becomes a medical and personal guide for that patient and an advocate for his or her health and well-being.

The MPCP model is an appealing contribution to medicine in general and psychosomatic medicine in particular. It keeps up the tradition of George Engel's bio-psycho-social approach, Michael Balint's understanding of the conscious and unconscious aspects of the doctor-patient relationship, and Viktor von Weizsäcker's patient-centered medicine. Moreover, it's a new and challenging field of work for those physicians (psychiatrists with psychosomatic subspecialization, family physicians or internists) who are interested in a 'holistic' bio-psycho-social understanding of illness, the subjectivity of the ill person within the complex influence of his or her milieu, as well as the intensive communication required in working with medical colleagues and other health care professionals. From my point of view, training in this model of care should be integrated in all psychiatric and primary care programs and fellowships.

However, the book goes far beyond the description of this new "MCPC" model. It offers an in-depth look at the problem of decision-making in medicine with a focus on physician-patient reciprocity. Because all medical treatments are collaborative undertakings, taking account of the subjectivity and inter-subjectivity of the patient's and the physician's experience is indispensable for creating a trusting doctor-patient-relationship and achieving effective clinical outcomes. In their approach, the authors meticulously describe the process of experience-based clinical judgment as a necessary contribution to evidence-based clinical strategy creation. In line with George Engel's appeal for 'looking inside and being scientific,'[1] they advocate a method for clinical accuracy through clinically useful and appropriate 'truing devices.' Such techniques can help the physician better understand and systematically assess the less tangible factors influencing the process of care.

Although this book should be required reading for the health care professional working with psychiatrically and medically comorbid patients, it is worthwhile reading for every physician with a deeper interest in the communication processes with patients as well as for the interested 'lay person'. It is noteworthy that the authors succeed in explaining their approach to complex problems using clear and comprehensible language. Further, it is a pleasure to read the case vignettes illustrating how the MPCP model works in moment to moment patient care.

Wolfgang Söllner, MD
Chief Physician, Klinikum Nürnberg Nord, Germany

---

[1] Engel G. The need for a new medical model: a challenge for biomedicine. Science. 1997;196:129–136.

Preface

The development of the medical–psychiatric coordinating physician model

I (Steven Frankel) began to develop this model over 20 years ago. My background is divided. As with many psychiatrists of my generation, in addition to psychiatric residency I undertook training and certification in psychoanalysis. I also became interested in developmental contributions to psychopathology and character, and, so, I became board certified in child and adolescent psychiatry. In clinical work with children and adolescents it is not possible to exclude from consideration the ongoing pathogenic influence of the environment, including parents, school, and culture.

At this point, from my practice and my role as a full-time faculty member at the University of Michigan Medical School, I was also becoming aware of the profound limitations of in-depth, interpersonal psychotherapy. Consequently, I began to write about the issue of personal change, change resulting from deliberately orchestrated interpersonal influence.

In short, I was continually propelled to develop a way of organizing treatment that encompassed all pertinent factors: biological, temperamental, psychological, environmental, and developmental. To be true to life none of these influences could be excluded from clinical consideration. To be operational, the model needed ways to prioritize contributing factors and select interventions. Algorithms, while quite useful, tend to be inflexible, not adaptable to multiple-factor situations where requirements constantly shift. This is, of course, always the case when the subjects under consideration are human beings.

In the years that followed, together with the counsel of Phil Erdberg, a great friend and a nationally prominent expert in tests and measures, I've written four books, each bringing the model forward, each with a subtitle containing the word "collaboration." Any complex clinical situation involving specialists of any sort requires useful communication and collaboration between all involved parties, patient and family included.

The move from a generic collaborative model to one centered around the integration of psychiatry and systemic medicine was natural. The interface between psychiatry and systemic medicine was a matter of personal interest and was a less popular topic at that time than it is now. So, that was the next area to tackle. Fortuitously, I found Jim Bourgeois through his excellent *Casebook of Psychosomatic Medicine* (Bourgeois *et al.*, 2008). For the past several years we've worked hard, along with Phil Erdberg, to refine this model and incorporate it into this book.

This background should give you an idea about why and how this model of care has come about. It should not be difficult to see why we picture this work as a potential subspecialization within psychiatry and as an ideal area of practice for psychiatrists who have training in psychosomatic medicine, or dual training in psychiatry and family practice or internal medicine. It also is promising as an area of practice for primary care physicians (PCPs) who are interested in undertaking some additional training to expand the range of their practice to address the needs of "complex patients," and especially those with psychiatric co-morbidity. These are the patients with systemic medical, psychiatric, and psychosocial co-morbidity who populate, and, in ways, drain the medical system.

In effect, these are the patients nobody wants. Their initial encounter is generally with primary care providers. Multiple referrals are made to specialists. Most frequently they are referred back to PCPs who may have neither the time, patience, nor the psychiatric skills to handle their incessant and often emotionally based complaints. These difficulties are often expressed as somatoform disorders or as physical accompaniments to mood and anxiety disorders.

Our proposal is as follows: that the healthcare system explicitly re-embrace these patients, through the vehicle of multidisciplinary teams, each structured to the needs of a specific patient or group of patients. Models for psychiatric and conjoined psychiatric-systemic medical care of these challenging patients have needed to be developed to encompass the practical realities surrounding their care. The medical–psychiatric coordinating physician (MPCP) model is designed for this purpose.

Endorsements

"Today, organized medicine struggles with the disorganized havoc that complicated patients routinely wreak on the efficiency of systematized, evidence-based, protocolized, ultimately simplistic practice approaches. Models that embrace complexity are needed. In a book richly embroidered with extended case studies, a trio of clinicians with decades of diverse experience among them formulate an approach to what they call the "psychiatrically comorbid, management-intensive complex patient." This model rests on the herculean shoulders of their version of the "compleat" doctor, the "Medical–psychiatric coordinating physician" (MPCP), a master of the medical, psychological, and diplomatic skills the authors contend are necessary to wrestle not only difficult patients, but also their befuddled treatment teams into clinically responsive submission. This model insists upon teamwork, with the MPCP as both head coach and cheerleader. For those of us laboring to make sense of the clinical maelstroms within which we spin – too often in isolation – this book offers ideas and reassurance to help master the storm rather than founder in its vortex. It provides a cerebral roadmap for overwhelmed and desparate clinicians striving to blaze sensible trails through senseless systems of care."

J. Michael Bostwick, MD, Professor of Psychiatry, Mayo Clinic, USA

"With this book, these experienced clinicians propose a very innovative model of clinical Medical–psychiatric work with complex patients. The MPCP model identifies, structures, and integrates the key elements needed to comprehensively understand the diagnostic and therapeutic aspects pertinent to efficiently and collaboratively approach a patient's Medical–psychiatric condition. Not only do the authors present the model, they also guide the reader step by step through the implementation process, its essential phases and pitfalls risks.

Throughout, the authors are clear and straightforward in addressing the clinical issues that clinicians must consider when working with all patients, particularly complex ones. These include patient bias, professional bias and subjectivity, and systemic/inter-professional work bias. So, it's a book on how to best evaluate and treat patients with all the complexities related to diagnostic and treatment issues. It considers the patient's medical and social conditions, most contemporary scientific knowledge, and the medical care environment.

In this time of fragmentation in the care of complex patients and "algorithmic practice," the MPCP Model addresses conflicting issues and offers patient-centered solutions. It also integrates aspects of shared decision-making and shared mental health care approaches. Some readers may be tempted to stop reading after a few chapters, finding the MPCP model too idealistic. I would invite you to read the book cover to cover, to better comprehend the model's realistic approach to patients care, and discover many pearls of clinical wisdom.

I most appreciated the author's efforts to increase clinical judgment through many "truing tools" presented and illustrated with numerous medical and psychiatric case vignettes. The model aims to facilitate the process of confirmation or rejection of clinical hypothesis, and improve clinical accuracy. The MPCP model will probably be recognized as an advantageous clinical–scientific model based on critical thinking, and a model offering a methodology for experienced based clinical judgment (EBCJ)."

Fabien Gagnon MD, DPsy, CCFP, CSPQ, FRCPC, FCFP, DFAPA, DFCPA, FAPM
Co-founder of the Canadian Academy of Psychosomatic Medicine, Professor,
Head of the Division of Consultation-Liaison Psychiatry and Psychosomatic Medicine,
Department of Psychiatry and Neurosciences, Université Laval, Québec, Canada

"Patients' trust is crucial to the outcome of medical treatment. This trust is often violated when treating patients with multi-morbidity as their treatment is complicated by all kinds of interactions, including diagnostic and pharmacological, reduced coping, and inconsistencies and inadequacies in communication among healthcare professionals. These factors are often ignored, negatively affecting the trust of patients and the outcome and cost of treatment.

This book focuses on the analysis and management of complexity, forming an antidote to the over-valuation and current dominance of the fragmenting DSM-IV, DSM-V classification. Thinking about complexity unifies the treatment of multimorbid patients and should serve as a guide to multi-disciplinary teams who treat these patients. Complexity thinking should be an essential part of training of these professionals, as it provides a unifying language which could unify the divided field of professional organizations focusing on multi-morbid patients. The value of this book for the further development of professional treatment of multi-morbid patients cannot be overestimated."

Frits J. Huyse MD, Professor, Department of Internal Medicine,
University Medical Center Groningen, The Netherlands

"Doctors Frankel, Bourgeois, and Erdberg's detailed and honest book deliberately exposes an embarrassing secret - that medical care in our society is unnecessarily divided. With decades of clinical experience each, they quietly encourage a revolution in the way we practice medicine. Why accept the artificial schism between mind and body when integration of care is so intuitive and effective? The "MPCP" model suggests that, rather than limiting ourselves by self-imposed boundaries, physicians, particularly psychiatrists, explore the full spectrum of a patient's mental and physical health, utilizing "truing" measures that enable us to judge our work by concrete results."

Debra Kahn, MD, Assistant Clinical Professor, Department of Psychiatry and Behavioral Sciences and Director, Psychosomatic Medicine Service, University of California at Davis, Sacramento, CA, USA

"This book proposes an innovative model for providing care for Medical–psychiatric complex patients, a rapidly growing population that require disproportionate attention and excessive resources for their care. According to this model, physicians, general psychiatrists, and physicians trained in both psychiatry and Internal/family medicine, lead multi-disciplinary teams and are accountable for efficiency and results. The physician-led "medical–psychiatric coordinating physician (MPCP)" model not only appears to improve treatment outcome, but also provides for containment of costs by reducing redundancy and curbing excess in the use of services. Other benefits include improved diagnostic accuracy and decision-making, as well as better communication among physicians and allied health professionals. This is a cutting-edge book, essential for medical educators, administrators, and providers."

Robert McCarron DO, Associate Professor, Department of Psychiatry and Behavioral Sciences, University of California at Davis, Sacramento, CA, USA

"Born from years of vigorous practice and conscientious reflection, this unique volume is a trusty trekking guide across clinical terrain that is both familiar and novel: familiar because the multi-dimensional challenges are recognized by every physician, yet novel because we are enabled to see old problems in fresh, invigorating relief. Do not let careful definitions or occasional new acronyms fool you: you are not holding an ivory tower treatise! This delightful work – suffused with rich, authentic clinical material (no idealized composite patients or mawkish bedside memoirs here) – grows on you. By the end, you have found a firm friend with whom you want to hike over and again. Rooted in high regard for the individual patient, tempered by real-life complexities, and unwilling to lose sight of evidence supported treatments, the authors generously give the Medical–psychiatric physician a strategy for transformative service that stimulates the mind and satisfies the soul."

Kemuel Philbrick, MD, Assistant Professor of Psychiatry, Mayo Clinic, USA

"This is a well-written guidebook for psychiatrists, primary care physicians, and students as they develop a way to consider and approach clinical work with complex cases. It has an engaging style using many well-timed case reports.

The authors articulate the need for coordination of care by a multidisciplinary physician team, bringing this topic of great current interest into focus by addressing the more difficult and complex patients with co-morbid medical and psychiatric conditions.

While the current movement towards team approaches applies to all patients, the complex patients addressed here are the ones that most require a care team. These prevalent patients represent the key problem every team effort must resolve because they are challenging, often refractory to current care, and have mental health problems. Implementing the patient centered, team-based approach outlined will enhance both care and safety for patients currently receiving uncoordinated care, responding to the concerns of the Institute of Medicine contending that modern medicine is derelict in patient-centered care and patient safety.

In addition, this book brings a very skilled and much needed psychiatric perspective to team care which can can guide non-mental health professionals in structuring their teams. Over two thirds of presently diagnosed (via epidemiological surveys) mental patients are never seen by mental health professionals, and are cared for entirely in primary care thirds by medical physicians who have had little training for this kind of work.

The professional and scholarly backgrounds of the authors are impeccable. This book will be germane and useful to ever-burgeoning numbers of providers, administrators, payors, and others interested in team-based care."

Robert Smith MD, Professor of Medicine and Psychiatry,
Michigan State University, East Lansing, MI, USA

"While clinics, research, teaching, and healthcare organization are still focused on specific diseases, physicians are increasingly confronted with complex patients suffering from multiple somatic and psychosocial morbidities. This book introduces a treatment model for diagnostically complex and management-intensive complex cases. The multiple interrelated dimensions of complexity – clinical, operational, diagnostic, and management complexity – and the rationale and clinical application of the proposed integrated treatment model are comprehensively described and discussed.

This very thoughtful book, written by clinicians for clinicians, will contribute to complex patients receiving better care, and help physicians to feel more at ease and better equipped to handle complex patients, a large patient population. This book should also be read by other healthcare professionals, such as researchers, teachers, or policy makers, who are motivated to help to deliver more adequate and efficient care to the complex medically ill."

Friedrich Stiefel, MD, Chief of Service, Psychiatric Liaison Service, University
Hospital of Lausanne, Switzerland

"If you're searching for a smarter, more effective way to take care of the 10% of patients who command 70% of our healthcare costs, this book is for you. The "complex patient" with co-morbid medical and psychiatric conditions demands a new approach and a new role for the psychiatrist leading the clinical care team. Here's a richly detailed guide to tackling one of healthcare reform's high priorities."

Lawson Wulsin, MD, Professor of Psychiatry and Family Medicine,
University of Cincinnati College of Medicine, Cincinnati, OH, USA

"Doctors Frankel, Bourgeois, and Erdberg propose an innovative model for providing individualized, comprehensive care for Medical–psychiatric complex patients–a group of "patients nobody wants." The MPCP model calls for psychiatrists to extend their duty as consultants to primary care providers, and become physician leaders who coordinate care among primary care providers, as well as, psychotherapists, social workers, and other medical and mental health specialists. This book uses case examples to illustrate the fact that, while some initial investment is needed to take care of the most complex Medical–psychiatric patients, in the long-run the investment pays off exponentially in terms of reduced, unnecessary medical work-ups, lower re-hospitalizations, and, most importantly, improved patient outcomes. The book is a must-read for medical educators, physical health and mental health policy makers, and physician leaders."

Glen Xiong, MD, Associate Clinical Professor, Department of Psychiatry and
Behavioral Sciences, University of California at Davis, Sacramento, CA, USA

Acknowledgments

Life is full of miracles. Mine have been manifold and go by the names of Diane Engelman, my remarkable neuropsychologist wife; Peter and Cara, my incomparable adult children; Tracy, Hilary, and Iishwara, the equivalent in the step-children category; and Kaliani and Jaidev, who top the "neatest grandchildren" list. All of these dear people have fueled my enthusiasm for developing the treatment model we describe in this book; a model of care that we hope will be welcomed as a significant contribution to our field.

And, then, of course, there is the inspiration of innumerable colleagues. Prominently included is Roger Kathol, MD, leader in the field of "clinical complexity," and an author for the forewords for this book. Special thanks go to Joanna Chamberlin, our editor at Cambridge University Press and an ever-present source of light and wisdom during the creation of this book, and to Richard Marley, Publishing Director for life sciences and medicine at Cambridge University Press, who discovered and encouraged us from the beginning.

Steven A. Frankel, MD

I wish to thank my supportive family: my wife, Kathleen M. Ayers, PsyD; my son Emile; and daughter Gigi for their support and encouragement.

Dr. Bourgeois wishes to dedicate his part of this work to the many inspirational leaders in Psychosomatic Medicine who serve as examples and role models for the integration of medicine and psychiatry. Their vision is one of unified medical care, especially pertinent for patients with "clinical complexity." This group of physicians is represented and supported by The Academy of Psychosomatic Medicine. "The Academy" has been in the forefront of the development of integrated models of care such as the one we present in this book. I hope that this volume serves as a significant support to patients, physicians, and other health professionals as they carry out this work.

James A. Bourgeois, OD, MD

For Judy and Danny.
Philip Erdberg, PhD

Complex treatments: the evolving place for a medical–psychiatric coordinating physician

Medicine has lost direction. You would have to look hard to find a patient, physician, or administrator who does not agree with the frustration reflected in that opinion. Managed-care and medical-center-based-clinic patients complain that their healthcare systems are too bureaucratized, their choices too limited, and the physicians they encounter more like "gatekeepers" than "healers." In the private practice, fee-for-service sector, the usual dissatisfaction is about the disorganization of services and lack of collaboration among physicians. Patients lament the fact that office visits have become unconscionably brief, medical treatment too impersonal, and that costs are escalating. Negotiating this fragmented system and its out-of-control expense can be maddening for both patient and physician (Kovner *et al.*, 2000; Gawande, 2007; Gawande *et al.*, 2009; Hussey *et al.*, 2009; Kovner, 2010).

With this book we hope to do our part to confront this dilemma. We intend to make our contribution at the clinical level, ultimately through the integrated treatment model we introduce in the following chapters. This method of patient care features a physician in a newly created role; that of the "Medical–Psychiatric Coordinating Physician" (throughout this book designated by *MPCP*). MPCP treatment is especially applicable for diagnostically complex and management-intensive *complex cases* (de Jonge *et al.*, 2006; Huyse *et al.*, 2006; Stiefel *et al.*, 2006; Latour *et al.*, 2007a; Leff *et al.*, 2009; Kathol *et al.*, 2010a; Grant *et al.*, 2011): those involving co-morbid systemic medical and psychiatric illnesses, and excessive utilization of resources, as well as requiring the participation of multiple interacting physician providers, healthcare workers, and consultants.

Throughout this book, while we spotlight this group of patients and develop the MPCP model, we also pay special attention to the essential complexity of clinical work ("clinical complexity") (Plsek & Greenhalgh, 2001), how it impacts the resolution of all the pathology we encounter, and how it can be best managed through the use of devices for improving clinical accuracy. We designate these techniques "truing measures," since they point the physician in the direction of technical precision and, ultimately, toward the best approximation of clinical "truth" (Campbell & Fiske,

1959; Arkes, 1981). We will elaborate on the use of truing devices throughout the book, especially as we discuss complex clinical cases. Regardless of the diagnostic or logistical considerations in a case, issues of *complexity* in clinical work and the requirement for the rigorous application of truing measures are never missing.

The responsibilities of the medical–psychiatric coordinating physician

We understand the MPCP as addressing two separate clinical dimensions. *Level 1*, the "microscopic," consists of individual physicians and other healthcare professionals rendering direct care and working within their own specialties. *Level 2*, the "macroscopic," refers to the multi-person system of interacting physicians and other health professionals that develops around each case. While working at *Level 1*, the physician strives for accuracy within clinical encounters using all the technical measures at his or her disposal.

While operating at *Level 2*, the MPCP coordinates and monitors the patient's overall treatment. From this vantage point the MPCP manages, optimizes, and, in effect, "treats" the patient's unified medical-psychosocial system, addressing its dysfunctions. He or she does this by leading a treatment team consisting of other physicians and allied healthcare professionals (Gittell *et al.*, 2000, 2008; Gittell, 2009). Communication of team decisions to the patient and, often, the patient's family members is central to this role. The MPCP's charge is to see that the team functions in a way that optimizes outcome. Overall, while most uniquely embracing the *Level 2* coordination role, the MPCP works alternately and, often, simultaneously, on *Level 1* and *Level 2*, taking on whatever tasks are required at each point to make the treatment most effective and applying truing measures to guide this work.

Levels of complexity represented in clinical work

As we move along in this book, our effort will be to explicate and keep track of multiple interrelated dimensions of complexity encountered in clinical practice and propose a model for dealing with these, while maintaining precision in our work. We have separated out the following four contributions to the *complexity* of clinical work and will take up each either directly or as we discuss cases. The two basic categories of complexity are designated by an asterisk. Examples of these categories are distributed throughout the book.

Categories of clinical complexity

**Clinical complexity*: the multiple considerations, either deliberate or spontaneously arrived at, that a clinician encounters when attempting to formulate and/or intervene in a case. "Clinical complexity," when it leads to the involvement of multiple participants, may predispose to "operational complexity."

Operational complexity: refers to a treatment effort involving multiple participants. These treatments generally benefit when those involved are organized as a treatment team.

Diagnostic complexity (a subcategory of clinical complexity): refers to the clinical entities, often co-morbid, that a clinician targets as he or she works with complex cases. Diagnostically complex patients are commonly encountered in medical services of major medical centers. An example would be a post-transplant patient who is also dependent on opioids or one with diabetes mellitus who suffers from Bipolar Disorder.

Management complexity (the extent to which management difficulties characterize a case): patients whose clinical management requirements are challenging. These patients are often referred to as "difficult" or "impossible" patients (they are often also "chronic"). They usually over-utilize resources and elude attempts to manage their care efficiently.

The clinical subpopulation being addressed

Having initiated the subject of complexity in clinical work and embarked on an initial exploration of its dimensions, we return to our ultimate interest, clinical implementation. Various models of care, apart from the MPCP model, have been proposed for the delivery of integrated psychiatric and systemic medical care for diagnostically and operationally complex outpatients (Katon *et al.*, 1995, 1996, 1999; Zatzick *et al.*, 2004; American College of Physicians, 2006; Wulsin *et al.*, 2006; Nutting, et. al, 2009; Kathol *et al.*, 2010a; Kates *et al.*, 2011; Katon & Unützer, 2011; Zatzick *et al.*, 2011).

Some of these care systems (Katon *et al.*, 1995, 1996; Zatzick *et al.*, 2004; Kathol & Gatteau, 2007; Kathol *et al.*, 2009, 2010b; Kates *et al.*, 2011; Katon & Unützer, 2011) endeavor to eliminate the familiar and, we believe, artificial, separation between the delivery of systemic medical and psychiatric services. In contrast to the reliance on physician leadership in the MPCP model, and often in the interest of cost effectiveness, treatment coordination in these treatments is generally accorded to non-physician case managers.

There is a sizable subgroup of these clinically and operationally, psychiatrically co-morbid, complex patients whose pathology, however, does not respond well to the care described by these models. The psychiatric illnesses of this group dominate the clinical picture (Kathol & Gatteau, 2007; Kathol *et al.*, 2009; Grant *et al.*, 2011), complicating and prolonging their treatments. For these patients it is especially desirable, and often imperative, to have a psychiatrist as MPCP. We designate this subpopulation "*Management-Intensive Patients*" and, in particular, "*Psychiatrically Co-morbid, Management-Intensive, Complex Patients.*"[1]

---

[1] It is noteworthy that an MPCP's role with this group is co-extensive with the work of psychiatrists with an interest in the interface of systemic medicine and psychiatry. It therefore may have special

When considering the future for the MPCP model for patient care, we also envision its coordinating features being embraced by interested PCPs. In that situation the MPCP model becomes simply the "Coordinating Physician Model." (As a parallel, see the statement edited by Norman B. Kahn [2004], corresponding author for the policy statement concerning "The future of family medicine," from the American Academy of Family Physicians.) Analogous to the charge of the MPCP, these treatments would be configured to suit the needs of difficult-to-diagnose-and-treat *management-intensive complex patients,* many of whom have failed in conventional treatments. However, the balance of their pathology would not be psychiatric. To assume this role these physicians would need additional training that includes the organization and direction of clinical situations with complex management responsibilities involving interrelated medical and psychosocial systems.

The fallacy of the mind–body divide

From this point we move to fundamental considerations relevant to the MPCP model: the integration of psychiatry and systemic medicine, as well as the nature of clinical reasoning that characterizes these two specialty areas.

We begin our exposition with a brief description of the intersection of psychiatry and systemic medicine. That aspect of complexity calls for additional attention as the diagnostic and operational requirements of the patient increase.

It is tempting but reductionistic to single out the "physical" and "psychiatric" manifestations of a disease process. Treatment in each sector is commonly allocated to specialists; e.g., internists for conditions that are primarily physical and psychiatrists for illness involving mental dysfunction. Nonetheless, these two areas almost always interrelate. Illness is generally experienced "wholistically," with a patient's personal and medical reality transcending Cartesian mind–body dualism.

In this book, through the MPCP-led model, we hope to reinforce the unity of objectives we believe prevails throughout general medicine and psychiatry. We hold that similarities and linkages between these areas are compelling. All physicians and allied health professionals seek the same goal: the biopsychosocial well-being of the patient. They use corresponding technology, including examinations, interviews, feedback from relevant external sources, and testing. As such, they perform complementary roles in the broad clinical enterprise. Throughout this book we will build on the similarities between psychiatrists and primary care physicians, analogies that can be understood along similar heuristic dimensions.

---

appeal to those trained in psychosomatic medicine or to "dual-trained" psychiatrists with additional qualification in internal medicine or family medicine. In the case of psychosomatic psychiatrists functioning as MPCPs, the PCP would continue to render much of the systemic medical care. Dual-trained psychiatrists can assume both roles. However, in either case the MPCP must assume overall direction of the work and actively monitor medical resource utilization.

Distinctions are useful, nonetheless. As such, we will employ the following definitions throughout this book. We will speak of "primary care," that is, internal medicine, family medicine, and pediatrics, as being mainly responsible for the management of *systemic* illness. These are illnesses that for the most part are not central nervous system (CNS)-based. Psychiatry typically deals with disorders of the CNS that are manifested as "*mental*" dysfunctions. Included in this category are disorders of cognition (e.g., dementia), mood (e.g., depression), anxiety (e.g., panic disorder), psychosis (e.g., schizophrenia), and social behavior (e.g., personality disorders).

The foregoing demarcation, however, does not precisely address CNS-based illnesses that involve areas of function that are more specifically "*physical*" than "*mental*," e.g., movement disorders and seizure disorders, and that are generally the province of neurology. Furthermore, whatever delineations prevail and are useful, many systemic illnesses have CNS-based, "*mental*" symptoms associated with their pathology or are co-morbid with discrete psychiatric disorders. Equally, it is not unusual for psychiatric illnesses to have associated systemic physical manifestations.

We return here to our delivery-of-care challenge. Guiding our project has been commitment to the dissolution rather than reinforcement of the "systemic medical versus psychiatry" division. We continue to address this issue through the vehicle of the MPCP-led model. Working within the MPCP-led model of care requires familiarity and competence with both sides of the mind–body Cartesian coin, as well a unified set of operational standards and medical objectives.

Unification

To illustrate our point about the essential unity between systemic medicine and psychiatry, let us consider two familiar chronic illnesses, one classically "systemic medical" and one "psychiatric."

From systemic medicine consider the following description of diabetes mellitus, its clinical presentation, and complications, as an example of these interdisciplinary linkages. This description is excerpted from the American Diabetes Association website, professional.diabetes.org, and from "Standards of medical care in diabetes – 2012" (American Diabetes Association, 2012).

Early signs of diabetes mellitus include: excessive thirst and increased fluid intake, extreme hunger, unusual weight loss, fatigue, irritability, & visual disturbance. Diabetes mellitus develops due to a diminished production of insulin (in type 1) or resistance to its effects (in type 2). Both lead to hyperglycemia which largely causes the acute signs of diabetes mellitus. Type 2 diabetes mellitus may go unnoticed for years because visible symptoms are typically mild, non-existent or sporadic, and usually there are no ketoacidotic episodes. Microangiopathy can cause one or more of the following: retinopathy, neuropathy, nephropathy, and cardiomyopathy. Macroangiopathy may lead to coronary artery disease, cerebrovascular disease, and peripheral vascular disease. Diabetes mellitus is often diagnosed when a patient suffers diabetic complications such as a heart attack, stroke, neuropathy, poor wound healing, visual impairment, fungal infections, or delivering a baby with macrosomia and/or hypoglycemia. Diagnosis is clinched by fasting plasma glucose level at or above 126 mg/dL (7.0 mmol/L), plasma glucose at or above 200 mg/dL (11.1 mmol/L) two hours after a 75 g oral glucose load as in a glucose tolerance test, symptoms of hyperglycemia and random plasma glucose at or above 200 mg/dL (11.1 mmol/L).

In psychiatry, formal diagnostic criteria are also quite exacting. Schizophrenia is an example. The following list of criteria is excerpted from the American Psychiatric Association's (2000) *Diagnostic and Statistical Manual*, version IV-TR (DSM-IV-TR).

Two or more of the following symptoms need to be present for much of the time during a one-month period (or less, if symptoms remitted with treatment). These include delusions, hallucinations, disorganized speech which is a manifestation of formal thought disorder, grossly disorganized (e.g., dressing inappropriately, crying frequently) or catatonic behavior. Other manifestations include negative symptoms; e.g., affective flattening, alogia, or avolition. If the delusions are bizarre, or hallucinations consist of hearing one voice participating in a running commentary of the patient's actions or of hearing two or more voices conversing with each other, only that symptom is required for diagnosis. The speech disorganization criterion is only met if it is severe enough to substantially impair communication.

The following evidence of social/occupational dysfunction needs to have been present for a significant portion of the time since the onset of the disturbance: deterioration to a point markedly below the level achieved prior to the onset in one or more major areas of functioning such as work, interpersonal relations, or self-care. Continuous signs of this aspect of the disturbance need to have persisted for at least six months. This six-month period must include at least one month of symptoms (or less, if symptoms remitted with treatment).

In addition, schizophrenia cannot be diagnosed if symptoms of a mood disorder or pervasive developmental disorder are present, or the symptoms are the direct result of a general medical condition or use of a substance, such as abuse of a drug or medication.

The scientific argument

We have considered two "prototypical" illnesses, one "systemic medical" and the other "psychiatric." Returning to points of intersection in the mind–body dichotomy, diabetes mellitus, in addition to the physical symptoms noted above, is well known to be associated with psychiatric co-morbidities such as depression, vascular dementia, and episodes of delirium during periods of systemic instability. In addition, the profound need for assertive medical self-management mandates that the treating physician keep close track of the patient's emotions and thinking, compliance with medical treatment, and capacity to tolerate the psychiatric burden of a chronically life-threatening and life-limiting illness.

By the same token, schizophrenia, while obviously "psychiatric" in its origins, is associated with high rates of smoking and its predicable systemic consequences. Obesity is a frequent metabolic consequence of many of the common psycho-pharmacological treatments used to treat it, and schizophrenia is associated with a 25-year reduction in life expectancy due to all causes. From a disease standpoint, then, one can understand diabetes mellitus as a "psychiatric" as well as a systemic illness, and schizophrenia as a "systemic" as well as a psychiatric illness.

Hopefully, you can see why we have gone to such trouble to bring the practices of general medicine and psychiatry into alignment. One focus rarely is adequate without the other. Primary care medicine patients often present with complicated personal histories, individual preferences, and temperamental differences that influence their ability to cope with illnesses. They exist in a social milieu that, as the examples in this book illustrate, may profoundly affect their ability to accept and work productively in treatment. Reciprocally, it almost goes without saying that psychiatric practice benefits from recognizing and taking on the more factual focus that characterizes the practices and standards that prevail in non-psychiatric medicine.

Shift here to the criteria for patient care and verification that prevail in general medicine. The components are actually quite straightforward. The physician is charged with finding out what is wrong with a patient, whether the primary etiology is biological, psychological, or environmental. To carry out this task he or she has the responsibility of coming up with a list of likely diagnoses and refining them through a careful process of elimination. Completing this process involves creating and implementing a treatment plan.

Finally, there is accountability. The physician is accountable for results, or, if these are short of the mark, for seeking additional information or consultation to discover why that is true and what to do about it. At this point the treatment plan may need to be modified or reformulated. We believe that these principles of care and verification are as relevant in psychiatry as in general internal medicine and family practice.

Medical treatment as a scientific project

We hold that the decision to undertake medical treatment involves the patient and physician in a one-subject scientific project. To clarify what we mean, the basis of any scientific undertaking can be summarized in the simple statement: Y is a function of X. Y is the dependent variable, in medicine the difficulty that brings the person into treatment. X represents independent variables, the factors $(X', X'',$ etc.) that together account for the patient's difficulty.

As an example, again consider the criteria for diagnosing diabetes mellitus. The patient's health is the dependent variable; the pathophysiology of the disease, as well as the patient's habits, are the independent variables. How and what the patient eats, and how well he or she can monitor blood glucose and follow through with medical instructions, are independent variables.

Switching to psychiatric practice, think of a patient with a social phobia or avoidant personality disorder who has difficulty establishing relationships. That is the dependent variable and our job is to discover all the independent variables – the Xs – that account for that difficulty. These factors might include family background, history of relationships, and temperament. If we could be clear about the identity of all the independent variables we would be able to solve the equation, making the Xs explain Y and reducing the "variance" associated with it. As a result we would be able to identify all the treatment interventions that might improve outcome.

By advocating for the identification and use of truing measures, the project we are embarking on has the goal of encouraging the physician to be as scientific as possible, striving to account for as many independent clinical variables as possible. By doing so, he or she should be in the best position to address the core clinical issues, the dependent variable(s), in each case.

Clinical judgment

Now to decision making: how physicians process all the data they have available to them into the sort of understanding that leads to effective interventions. Physicians make decisions, literally hundreds of them during every office visit. These are usually small decisions that "microscopically" dictate the course of a treatment. While almost all of these choices require some deliberation, many are relatively spontaneous. As such, most involve a good measure of "clinical judgment" (Goldberg & Werts, 1966; Arkes, 1981; Downie & Mcnaughton, 2000; White & Stancombe, 2003).

Clinical judgment has both objective and subjective components. Included in the influences – the independent variables – shaping these judgments are the clinician's training, his or her currency with recent developments in the field, and clinical experience. Added, are sources of data that are technically specific, including clinical interviews and examinations, laboratory and imaging studies, and information from collateral sources. For gauging outcome the physician also has standardized tests and rating instruments at hand. Subjective contributions to this process include the clinician's common sense, personal capacity for organizing and prioritizing clinical data, personal opinions, and prejudices. Thus far only the clinician's contribution has been mentioned. However, there are actually few applications of clinical judgment that are not colored by the patient's preferences and mood.

Clearly it is impossible to remove the human substrate from clinical work. It should be obvious, then, that clinical judgment exists in *partnership* with but is *distinct from* the technical factors contributing to clinical decision making. The "data" clinicians deal with are always commingled with interpretation and opinion. The physician is the main author of these judgments, but the patient's opinion and reactions influence them as well.

Strategy: orchestrating clinical judgment

Orchestrating treatment introduces multiple levels of complexity, extensive sources of variance, into the clinical encounter. Beginning with the available data and using his or her judgment, the physician settles on a series of actions. There are major actions and minor ones. Some of the resulting strategies are consciously worked out in the clinician's mind; others are more spontaneous but no less complex. Together, these actions constitute one segment of a broader clinical strategy. The following are two examples.

Stanley

Stanley, a 62-year-old patient who had three spinal surgeries and multiple psychotherapies, was referred to me, SAF, for assessment and treatment of his psychiatric and neurological illness. While he had been accorded multiple psychiatric diagnoses generally ranging from anxiety to depressive disorders, the one that seemed most applicable was "Cyclothymic Disorder," a diagnostic category indicative of a mood disorder and categorized in the DSM-IV-TR under "Bipolar Disorders." Stanley had just moved to a location near my office, and as a result had to give up his psychiatrist of five years. Stanley was aware that the psychiatric treatment was going to end sooner or later anyway, since the psychiatrist was being treated for end-stage multiple sclerosis. From the very beginning, according to Stanley everything I did was "wrong." My office was "too hard to find," the picture on my website led Stanley to expect me to be younger, and, to make matters worse, when Stanley missed his second appointment I charged him for it. That Stanley had never bothered to cancel the appointment apparently didn't count. Stanley's argument, after the fact, was that his wife had a "personal emergency" at the time of the appointment, making it hard for him to pay attention to his own obligations.

In part out of my personal loyalty to his previous psychiatrist, I hung in with Stanley. I hypothesized that his vociferous complaints mainly represented a displacement of disappointment and anger about losing her, and were not primarily being instigated from within our relationship. Since she was terminally ill, I assumed that Stanley could not allow himself to acknowledge his anger at her. My clinical judgment, my clinical strategy as it developed, was at least in part based on guesswork. In this instance it paid off. Stanley's anger abated, we discussed his frustration, and then could refocus on his clinical problems.

Once treatment was established, I discovered that Stanley was in excruciating pain. According to him, no previous surgery had brought relief. "Can you help me Dr. Frankel? No one else has been able to. They are all a bunch of quacks. My god does it hurts [as he squirmed]!" While my first strategic move had worked, the next had to be more deliberate. I said I would continue to work with him but that I needed to contact his other physicians and get more information. Two weeks later, after I spoke to the orthopedic surgeon who had last operated on Stanley's back (why not a neurosurgeon, I wondered?), and talked at length to the pain specialist with whom Stanley had worked, I was better armed. I had been informed by the orthopedic surgeon that in her opinion no additional surgical procedure was likely to help Stanley. But, that opinion came from an orthopedist, not a neurosurgeon. I also realized that Stanley was dependent on oxycodone as well as a number of other medications affecting his central nervous system, all of which he was taking daily as a complex medication "cocktail."

My fact finding was beginning to pay off. Clearly Stanley had not been apprised of all the options available to him, and, perhaps because of a lack of coordination among his physicians, his medical situation was being suboptimally managed. My clinical strategy was deliberate and evolved as treatment went along. My next move was to reassemble Stanley's physicians into a formal treatment team and establish a "network" so that we could communicate and work together. I informed them that I was doing this and, after Stanley agreed that it was a good idea, created a plan for our collaborative work. As we move throughout this book we will continue to develop this model, *the medical–psychiatric coordinating physician* model, for coordinated practice with complex cases. As already noted, the MPCP assembles, leads, and manages a treatment team, making sure goals are consistent, team members in synchrony, and clinical outcome monitored

Roberta

Our next case Roberta involves a prototypical but "difficult" to manage psychiatric patient, with a diagnosis of Bipolar II Disorder, most recent episode Depressed. We have included it to illustrate the central place of clinical judgment when dealing with psychiatric aspects of difficult treatments. The systemic medical aspects of the case were elusive since the abdominal and chest pain frequently reported by the patient were never shown to have any systemic medical basis. In addition to her PCP, multiple medical specialists had been consulted over a period of years. For the treatment of her psychiatric symptoms the patient was receiving therapeutic doses of bupropion and lamotrigine. She had been hospitalized five years earlier after a suicide attempt, was 46 years old at the time of referral, and was referred because she was having trouble in the workplace.

Clinical dilemma
Imagine yourself as the patient's psychiatrist. As you meet with her you discover that she is probably about to get herself into major trouble by triggering a crisis at work. As you see it, this propensity is likely associated with her bipolar mood instability. Making matters worse, her medical complaints have escalated, causing frequent absences from work. She is "infuriated" with her boss, and wants to file a complaint alleging workplace abuse. You decide to confront her with the potential problematic consequences of her planned behavior. However, through experience with her you are aware that directly challenging this patient is itself likely to incite anger and be disruptive to treatment.

What to do in this situation? Here are the major considerations. (1) The strongest is her sense of injury at work and fury at her boss. Accordingly, her physical complaints have escalated, causing her to miss work on several occasions over the past month. (2) Second, based on past experiences with her, you know she has difficulty controlling herself when emotionally overwrought. (3) Available, however, is her demonstrated ability to think things through if given sympathetic guidance. (4) You also know that she tends to perform well in her job, at least when her mood is not contaminated by anger.

Judgment

Now turn to the judgment I (SAF) used in my work as the treating psychiatrist. I told the patient I "understood" and could empathize with her sense of injustice, but also cautioned her to reflect on her intended actions since I was "clear that she didn't want to lose her job." I then made suggestions about how she might safely and effectively approach this situation, commenting on her "usual excellent ability to think things through." Here is where I also brought in pertinent experiences from earlier in her life, recognizing their probable contribution to her rage at her boss. Throughout her childhood her mother did little other than criticize her, constantly inciting anger that was never worked through. I asked her whether there might be parallels between those childhood experiences and her current problems with her female boss.

However, more fundamentally, I was aware that the patient's rage was likely to be mitigated by empathy in the form of concerned advice paired with specific suggestions about how she might better manage her work situation. I further reasoned that attention to her current medical complaints and being in touch with her PCP and gastroenterologist would underscore that I was taking her seriously.

And, then, one more piece of strategy, with the aim of additionally consolidating the treatment alliance. Since my suggestions were likely to be weak against her powerful emotions, I decided to offer the patient additional support by calling her between appointments. Clinical judgment was instrumental in guiding me at each step in this process.

Strategy

As is illustrated in this case, clinical strategy is the end product of clinical judgment. But, it also involves calculations of risk. If I do "A" then "X" is likely to occur. However, if I do "B" the probable outcome is "Y." Arriving at these judgments often requires implementing small trials of the strategy. Informal attempts of treatment strategy paired with feedback are one of the "truing" activities described throughout this book. Once you initiate these trials, and if you discover your strategy is off the mark, you can sharpen your focus by bringing in one or more additional truing measures such as getting additional laboratory tests or taking a more targeted and detailed history.

As noted earlier, truing devices are techniques through which physicians and other healthcare professionals can improve and track the accuracy of their work, thereby "tightening" the clinical process. As in our example, revisions of strategy tend to happen spontaneously as treatment evolves, often as a result of a collaborative, verbal or non-verbal exchange between the patient and physician. This kind of patient–physician collaboration is one more of the many truing devices we will discuss throughout the book.

Options

Return to our patient and you, as the treating psychiatrist. There are several additional interventions you could consider at this point. For example, further pharmacological treatment is probably desirable. Also, the last described intervention, calling her between meetings, could be expanded by bringing in family members. You have a suspicion that meetings with the patient's husband and perhaps even her children might be seen by her as supportive. You also know that the patient has been talking about changing careers. She is unclear, however, about how to evaluate this possible objective and has worried about its advisability. Measured support from you for discussing this issue might also be welcomed by her.

Treatment team

Here, we find ourselves faced with a situation where switching to a formal treatment team structure might well enhance the management of the case. Clearly that team would include her PCP and current medical specialists. Also, think about how much stronger your work might be if family members were intermittently available for collaboration and a vocational counselor could be added to the team. According to this plan you would remain in the role of both the psychiatrist and treatment coordinator. As the team is created, a revised treatment plan would be developed by yourself in collaboration with the team and the patient.

Afterthought

An important point here is that clinical work continually requires the infusion of clinical judgment and is always emphatically strategic. It is unusual for a clinical strategy to remain uncomplicated and fixed over time, measures representing new independent variables being called for and existing ones shifting in importance. Physicians are confronted with this reality daily. Patients hear what their physicians recommend but regularly fail to comply, afterwards claiming they haven't received the care they need. That this complexity, representing multiple sources of variance, is characteristic of all clinical practice would be hard to discern from basic texts on internal medicine or psychiatry. The literature frequently makes it sound like clinical principles and their implementation are a relatively sure thing, an established system of theory and practice a physician can depend on as she or he works with a patient. In contrast, experienced physicians know that, "on the firing line," the work is rarely so clear and certain. If you, as a physician, don't bend as clinical requirements change, you will be soon be boxed in (or out), trapped by theory and practice guidelines. There may be little room for exercising judgment about how to manage the inevitable idiosyncratic developments.

Truing

So, how, given the place of opinion and subjectivity in clinical work, does a physician actually stay on course? How does he or she know the next best move for achieving results? And, how can he or she be certain that these are likely to be most favorable? Here, again, is where truing comes in. Repeating the definition, "truing" refers to devices, personal and formal, that are used to move clinical work ever closer to "truth." These measures account for "variance" inherent in a clinical procedure (Borum *et al.*, 1993). Conviction about the accuracy of the clinical process and the patient's requirements is progressively arrived at by using successive truing measures, incrementally consolidating one's certainty about the accuracy of clinical measurements through a series of "successive approximations," a notion similar to the mathematical concept of "asymptote" (Abelson, 1985). But, since the "truth" of a clinical impression must always at least partially elude us, support for the value of a truing sequence ultimately rests on obtaining measurable results (Aron, 1991, 1992, 1996; Hoffman, 1998). Hence, *results that can be defined, measured, and compared to a standard specified as a desirable outcome for that piece of work* is our version of "clinical truth," and will remain so throughout the book.

Approaches to truing

Truing devices commonly used in practice include the following.
(1) Physician variables, such as training and experience.
(2) Background and empirical data from the patient, gained through interviews and serial clinical examinations.
(3) Records of past treatments and hospitalizations.
(4) Interviews with collateral sources of information such as family members, previous physicians, and other professionals.
(5) Diagnostic tools:
    (a) the clinical interview and examination, repeated as required;
    (b) self-report instruments, including check lists completed by the patient, physician, or both;
    (c) laboratory and diagnostic imaging findings;
    (d) psychologist-administered psychometric tests.
(6) Ongoing correctives:
    (a) physician self-evaluation; for example, using the *Self-Other Rapid Assessment Method* described in Chapters 4 and 5, reviews of relevant literature, and consultations with colleagues;

    (b) moment-to-moment collaboration between patient and physician, each regularly providing feedback to the other.

(7) The findings from trial periods of treatment strategy.

(8) Monitoring of treatment progress and outcome, using:
    (a) check lists
    (b) self-report assessment instruments
    (c) laboratory and diagnostic imaging findings
    (d) psychologist-administered psychometric tests
    (e) formal outcome measures specific to that treatment.

(9) Intermittent reports specifying treatment progress and updates to the treatment plan. These may be written or verbal. They are created by the physician or MPCP in a team-led treatment and revised through collaborative feedback from the patient.

(10) The intersection and repetition of multiple truing measures, allowing for both confirmation and contradiction of clinical judgment through "successive approximations" and potentially generating new truing measures unique to that treatment.

(11) Add to this list truing devices used specifically by the MPCP for maintaining the accuracy of work at the team level. These will be spelled out in subsequent chapters.

Most chapters in this book expand upon one or more of the named truing devices.

Subjectivity, the bottom line in clinical work

This topic has been our silent partner throughout this chapter. The ground that clinical judgment and strategy are built on is indeed boggy. Orienting factors such as clinical experience and training lend an air of objectivity to what a physician does. But, this apparent certainty rarely tells the whole story.

Return to Stanley

Stanley is a good example. I (SAF) had seen lots of Stanleys over the years. They are always finding fault with their physicians, ultimately burning them out. Their self-management of pain and coping capacity is almost non-existent. They tend to be volatile.

The description here starts just after Stanley was referred to me. The clinical findings were reasonably straightforward. In Stanley's case, his orthopedic surgeons had actually seen his spinal pathology when they operated on him. They knew its relevant features. What was less clear, at least from my standpoint, was whether they may have made a mistake by not turning the case over to a neurosurgeon. Stanley had also irritated them, and the last thing they wanted to do was spend more time dealing with his complaints. In the end they "silenced"

Stanley with opioids and sedation. You can see how the ground was disappearing from beneath my feet, even at the beginning of my work with Stanley.

But, it gets worse. I (SAF) quickly began to respond to Stanley the way all the other physicians did. Honestly, after a few weeks of seeing him, I just wanted him to leave or at least shut up. As you may remember from the description earlier in this chapter, Stanley came into my office ready to fight. The clinical findings were one thing. Stanley's reaction to his medical problems and our reaction to each other were another. The likelihood that I, his pain medicine specialist, and his surgeons could see clearly enough to find an alternative medical or surgical plan was curtailed by our preconceptions and reactions to Stanley. And, while none of us really wanted to work with Stanley, it went both ways. He had limited patience for us, as well. Constructively dealing with the subjective influences in this treatment made the ground on which we walked very boggy indeed.

Physician's annoyance

Stanley's story applies equally well in most areas of clinical practice and highlights the topic of how subjectivity may afflict our work. Another clinical example follows. Simply substitute "chronic, non-specific medical complaints" or "multiple unexplained symptoms" for the psychiatric illness and idiosyncrasies affecting a patient, and you have this new patient, perhaps the third one who walked into your office yesterday. You have seen plenty of patients like this one. His self-confidence is flimsy and he insists that you take everything he says quite literally. But, something about his demeanor irritates you. He never stops wanting to tell you the details of his every symptom during the past week, always making it impossible to get to a productive "clinical focus." Even worse, when one medical symptom disappears there are always two more to take its place.

You decide to try a behavioral measure, tracking the patient's complaints and relating each to his core concerns; in this case, fear of aging and death. You determine that at each visit you and the patient will formally track these concerns and the patient's progress in dealing with them. As new data become available, you can collaboratively revise the treatment goals and the steps for achieving them. Your experience with similar patients suggests that with these behavioral measures in place the patient may relent and be able to work in a more focused way. But, that doesn't happen, and when you see the patient again he just keeps talking about trivial matters.

This turn of events is irritating to you. Nonetheless, you as his psychiatrist or primary care physician stay steady and force yourself to remain attentive. Yet, the patient picks up on your irritation. He communicates, both silently and in words, his suspicion that you are becoming annoyed with him. In response, even though you know that these allegations are accurate, you continue to hide your reactions and maintain an affirmative demeanor. The result, however, is that treatment rapport begins to erode. The patient grows distant and begins to miss appointments.

Here's where objectivity goes out the window and subjectivity comes in. From your training and clinical experience you were aware of the potential consequences of communicating annoyance to a patient. While you weren't overt about it, something about your reaction must have been communicated to him; perhaps through your tone of voice. In this situation, however, you were quite sure that the patient understood what you were asking for clinically. In your view, he just could not stay the course.

Of course, you knew that your reactions and the patient's would be partially based on personality factors like temperament and that a mismatch could cause problems. It is no surprise to you that you evoked stereotyped reactions in each other. But neither of you were consciously aware that the involved factors were so seriously contaminating the work until after that happened. Neither of you meant to be provoked or were even aware of your levels of annoyance. That feeling state, subliminal irritation and the shared lack of awareness of it, is what we mean by subjectivity. We are referring to the fundamental, visceral level of our experience as physicians, the dimension that exists beyond conscious knowing. This factor underpins and makes uncertain every clinical encounter.

To reiterate: clinical judgment, clinical experience, and the strategies physicians come up with frequently lead to successful clinical actions. The diabetes is under better control. Depression improves. Social isolation resolves. Truing helps make the clinical process more certain. But, what none of these considerations accounts for are the person-specific variables. No one, no psychiatrist, primary care physician, psychotherapist, or friend, knows another person well enough to be certain of exactly how that person will deal with an illness, or what interpersonal response that person will come up with. Illnesses and people change from moment to moment and day to day. So, we are again on the shaky ground that makes medical and personal situations so uncertain, and, thus, so interesting.

How often has a patient come to you after visiting several physicians, some of whom you know and respect, and told you they were inadequate? How many times have you encountered a person who is lost and confused because their spouse of 25 years left them without notice? Typically the story continues with, "But we knew each other so well..."

What to do now

Here we return to our original premise: that all clinical work, whether in psychiatry or systemic medicine, needs to adhere to the principles and standards that govern good medical treatment. These principles include:

(1) Careful attention needs to be paid to developing a working diagnosis and formulating a treatment plan (Faraone & Tsuang, 1994; White & Stancombe, 2003).
(2) Applying the truing measures we have listed is probably the surest way to achieve an acceptable outcome.

(3) The treatment should be monitored to make sure progress is occurring.

(4) Over time, it is likely that the treatment plan will have to be revised in accordance with changes in the patient's clinical condition and life circumstances.

(5) The adequacy and significance of the observed changes are assessed by reference to outcome measures established at the beginning of treatment and revised over time.

Consistently, throughout this book, we introduce another, entirely different, kind of truing provision: one that makes use of people other than the physician and patient who are collaborators in, or consultants to, the treatment. In primary care medicine these people generally are other medical specialists. In psychiatry, apart from other specialized physicians, consultation may be obtained from allied health professionals. On the personal side, family members may have a profound influence on the course and success of the treatment and can, and often should, be engaged as informants or participants in the management of the treatment.

Clinical work in this circumstance becomes most usefully organized around a treatment team. The leader of this team convenes and coordinates the treatment, making sure that it stays on course over time. Given how frequently these cases include complex psychiatric and systemic medical co-morbidity, we hold that this coordinating person should be a physician, a psychiatrist when, as is typical with clinically and operationally complex cases, psychiatric co-morbidity is prominent. Further supporting the value of psychiatric training and experience for an MPCP is the requirement for understanding the psychology and logistics of team coordination, work with families, and the ubiquitous psychiatric, psychological, and social difficulties with which these types of patients present. An MPCP's training and experience provides that person with the skills to understand and prioritize these clinical issues, as well as organize and coordinate other physicians and allied health professionals.

The treatments most appropriate for MPCP-led care were described at the beginning of the chapter as involving a "multi-person system of interacting physicians and other medical professionals." In addition to physicians, allied health professionals, and at times more than one care delivery system, the cooperative input of the patient and family members is likely to be pertinent to the work.

The notion of a "complex case" and its treatment will be elaborated throughout this book. Here is a summary of the definition with which we will be working.

A common use of the term "complex case" in the medical literature implies systemic medical–psychiatric co-morbidity (de Jonge *et al.*, 2006; Stiefel *et al.*, 2006; Kathol & Gatteau, 2007; Safford *et al.*, 2007; Kathol *et al.*, 2010a; Grant *et al.*, 2011). In some situations this designation refers to the psychiatric co-morbidity that follows difficulty coping with systemic illness, although in others this relationship is reversed and the systemic illness is exacerbated by psychiatric illness. Examples of patients with significant systemic medical–psychiatric co-morbidity include those with difficulty managing organ transplantation and coexisting substance use disorders or depression, and patients with disabling somatic complaints for which there are little or no objective physical, laboratory, or diagnostic imaging findings.

In this book, we broaden the use of the term "complex case" to include operational and management complexity. By making this shift we are able to encompass an expanded range of cases that make use of the MPCP's particular skills for sorting among, coordinating, and managing challenging clinical presentations.

We hold to this definition and, as well, further identify a subgroup of patients we feel is particularly appropriate for MPCP treatment.[2] These patients are difficult to manage, do not respond well to conventional care, and over-utilize personnel and resources. As mentioned previously, we call this group: "*management intensive, complex patients*," or – more precisely – "*psychiatrically co-morbid, management-intensive, complex patients*," the psychiatric aspect of their illness and management issues dominating.

The MPCP, as we conceive of this role for dealing with complex patients, then, should be a physician, and in the case of the types of patients we describe in this book, a psychiatrist, experienced in work with co-morbid psychiatric and systemic medical illness. He or she takes responsibility for organizing, managing, and following the diagnostic and operational complexities of a treatment. To this end she or he creates and coordinates a treatment team, making sure the team works effectively in producing the best possible results. If the treatment goals turn out not to be achievable, the MPCP then works with team members to come up with revised clinical strategies and outcome measures, or, in some cases, with an alternative treatment plan. We will say a good deal more about the MPCP throughout the following chapters.

---

[2] These patients are a subgroup of the broader population of "complex patients." By definition the broad group of complex patients have co-morbid systemic medical and psychiatric illnesses, use resources excessively, and require the participation of multiple interacting physician providers, healthcare workers, and consultants for their care.

Addendum for Chapter 1

"Clinical complexity" further elaborated

When looked at closely, clinical work is astonishingly complex and requires elaboration beyond that already given. We are referring to the multiple determinants that shape a diagnostic formulation and treatment plan (Tables 1.1 and 1.2) and the way we come to our moment-to-moment decisions about how to treat.

There are at least two primary sources of *clinical complexity* (Table 1.1). The first, which we will call "*inherent complexity*," reflects the general, descriptive variables selected to define the case and the assortment of personal and interpersonal factors always at work in clinical situations. The second, "technical complexity," consists of the mixture of diagnostic considerations specific to the case, whether psychiatric, systemic medical, or psychological.

Let's consider exactly what we mean when we talk about "a case." Here are some possible variables, each associated with "inherent complexity." In framing a case we may primarily be referring to (1) the patient and his or her systemic medical issues, as well as his or her personal psychology and psychopathology ("this is a previously well-adjusted, 34-year-old depressed man ..."). Instead (Table 1.2), we may want to invoke a more comprehensive perspective that includes (2) psychological and sociological factors impacting the patient beyond his or her personal psychology, and incorporating, for example, the patient's family and cultural background. We may also elect to add (3) the care systems within which the patient is being treated ("this is a case of a recently hospitalized ..."; "this is a case being managed collaboratively by ..."). In addition, we may decide to focus on the patient's prognosis and its (4) near-term status, as in the situation, for example, of a hospitalized patient, or, alternatively, the longer view, as one would have with an office-based or clinic-based outpatient.

Table 1.1 Dimensions of clinical complexity

"Inherent" Clinical Complexity (some out of many possible defining categories are listed below)	"Technical" Clinical Complexity	Extra-Treatment Factors that Add to Clinical Complexity
Patient: descriptive parameters e.g., age, socioeconomic status	Psychiatric diagnoses	Family configuration
Treatment-specific parameters: (1) type of treatment, (2) location of treatment e.g., outpatient, (3) intended length of treatment, (4) etc.	Systemic medical diagnoses	Occupation
The assortment of personal and interpersonal factors influencing treatment	Psychological and psychosocial factors influencing treatment	Cultural influences
Resources available to support treatment		

From there we move to another source of "inherent complexity": that associated with the imperfections of the clinical process. When looked at closely, clinical work can, and often does, lack (5) technical, e.g. diagnostic, clarity (e.g., what exactly do we mean when we say someone suffers from "major depression," or "needs supportive care?") and can easily be confounded by (6) imprecise communication between involved clinicians, as well as between these clinicians and the patient.

Finally, when several clinicians are involved in the case (in the text we call this category "operational complexity"), there may be (7) incompatibilities between the points of view and procedures each introduces, and their judgments about how and when to act.

Note, of course, that every case – even if its parameters are clearly spelled out – is (8) susceptible to multiple diagnostic designations and case formulations, each one subject to assumptions deriving from the involved clinician's training and personal biases.

So, "a case" is likely to mean different things to different people, each clinician's take also influenced by a multitude of person-specific factors including his or her specialty, clinical training, clinical experience, and personal psychology and preferences.

The product of all these "inherent" sources of complexity is the dissimilarity in strategies separate clinicians would come up with if they attempted to work with the same patient. We have already classified several types of "inherent complexity." As we go on to discuss the following case we bring in "*technical complexity*," the challenges when the patient presents with a confounding mixture of diagnostic issues.

Table 1.2 Some components of "a case": determinants that define the case and influence its management (each line reads from left to right)

Basic categories	Spouse	Children	Others
Personal psychology of patient			
Personal psychopathology of patient			
Psychology and psychopathology of other key participants			
Systemic medical considerations			
Family	Spouse	Children	Others
Organization of case (basic types)	Informal: communication between providers based solely on clinical need	Formal, Variation #1: each provider with designated duties but no case coordinator	Formal, Variation #2: treatment team with coordinator
Care systems	Outpatient/office based	Clinic/hospital based	
Time frame (i.e., prognosis) for care	Care limited to acute problem	"Stepped care" (Katon et al., 1999)	Protracted treatment with single provider
Technical clarity of case formulation, e.g., diagnostic clarity; how are parameters of case determined?	Methods used: formal	Methods used: observational	
Precision of communication between team members; with patient and family	Methods used for communication: telephone, email, EMR	Provisions for communication between providers, e.g., telephone, email, EMR	
Compatibility between providers and agreement between them about their recommendations	Number and identity of providers (e.g., their specialties)		
Multiplicity of diagnoses and case formulations			
Physicians' training, clinical experience, technical orientation			

EMR = electronic medical record.

Case example illustrating "Technical Complexity"

Consider Randy, an 18-year-old patient who survived a serious head injury followed by coma at age 6. Complicating her clinical course were disfiguring facial lacerations and fractures requiring extensive repair. Several years later, presumably in part as a result of her early medical trauma, she presented with anorexia nervosa and a conduct disorder focused around risk-taking, and including substance abuse and sexual promiscuity. I (SAF) was originally called in to provide treatment for her multiple psychiatric disorders.

The first order of clinical business was medical, working with Randy's primary care physician to deal with the psychological and systemic medical consequences of Randy's by now life-threatening eating disorder. The major responsibility for monitoring her entire medical condition, however, was soon mine, since Randy generally refused to cooperate with any of the adults in her life, including physicians.

The second involved focusing squarely on the psychology and management of Randy's substance use disorder and rebelliousness. Overall, the clinician now coordinating her care, myself, needed to create a treatment team that could respond to all facets of Randy's medical and psychiatric needs.

However, Randy insisted on doing things in her own way. Soon after I became involved in her care, she abruptly moved in with her boyfriend, cut off regular communication with her parents, and throughout this time neglected her doctors' cautions about the life-threatening nature of her disease. She simply "didn't want to hear" the facts.

In addition to interpersonal negotiation with Randy, working effectively with her behavior and disease processes required strict coordination between her internist, a dietician who specialized in eating disorders, and her divorced parents. Also available was a psychologist who performed a psychometric personality assessment in order to get a clearer picture of the nature and extent of Randy's psychopathology. In spite of her parents' and physicians' insistence, Randy was unwilling to enroll in a rehabilitation program for substance abuse or consider hospitalization for treatment of her active and progressing eating disorder.

Shift back for a moment from "technical" (Randy's systemic medical problems and psychopathology) to "inherent" complexity. In cases like this, coordination among professionals, and between them and the patient and family, frequently isn't easy (the subcategory of "inherent complexity" being referred to is "Operational complexity," described at the beginning of Chapter 1 under the heading "Levels of complexity represented in clinical work").

Managing and repairing disruptions in treatment is always the responsibility of the team coordinator. Here are two examples from our work with Randy. On one occasion Randy's parents failed to alert the rest of the treatment team that Randy had disappeared for a week and had reappeared only when she required emergency medical care. A similar disruption in the team's effort occurred when Randy's always angry mother skipped two consecutive family therapy meetings and brought Randy instead to an alternative medicine practitioner who wanted to treat her anorexia nervosa with natural remedies. This episode, for a second time, led to a trip to the emergency room; this time by ambulance. At the emergency room she was catechetic (weighing 43 kg, height 1.63 m [95 pounds, height 64″]), had poor skin turgor, and some hair loss and the proliferation of lanugo. Her physical exam revealed sinus bradycardia and orthostatic hypotension; the electrocardiogram (ECG) showed QTc prolongation. She was moderately anemic, while her electrolytes were within normal limits. She was admitted for medical hospitalization, but, a week later, refused transfer to an eating-disorders unit.

Meanwhile, my problems engaging Randy continued. She perceived me as the doctor who brought only news about what she shouldn't do. As Randy saw it, her job was to resist. Our treatment alliance was tenuous and needed constant repair.

When designing a treatment, "inherent complexity" is always there framing the boundaries and requirements of the case. Like Randy, many patients with difficult-to-treat medical or psychiatric pathology are also "technically complex." Reflecting this aspect of complexity, their treatment may require the collaborative involvement of multiple physicians and healthcare professionals.

And, the bottom line? We believe that to reduce the multiple sources of variance (inherent complexity plus technical complexity) in a clinical process, coordination between involved professionals, as well as between these people and the patient, is mandatory. This perspective is the starting point for understanding our MPCP team treatment model. If an individual practitioner rather than a multi-professional team, for example, a primary care physician or a psychiatrist alone, had assumed Randy's care, things might have turned out quite differently. It is likely that each clinician's treatment would have been narrowly formulated, evolved through the lens of his or her own specialty. Missing would have been the checks and balances inherent in a collaborative, team-focused model. While Randy's treatment was challenging and disorderly enough to make it difficult for a team of specialists to handle, it is hard to imagine a single practitioner having successfully managed it.

The MPCP treatment team method of patient care is intended to address the fragmentation in the care for the complex patients referred to earlier in this chapter. Because of the excessive demands these patients make, as well as the multiplicity of professionals who inevitably become involved in their care, their treatments tend to be loosely structured and lacking in organization. Administrative and intra-team difficulties frequently confound these efforts.

The MPCP model addresses these issues through case and team management, beginning with an initial comprehensive evaluation and then reassessments as treatment evolves. The MPCP, the physician who heads the treatment team, works collaboratively with all team members, as well as monitors their interactions with the patient and family. The MPCP assembles, leads, and coordinates each case, organizing and directing the multidisciplinary treatment teams required for the management of these patients. He or she establishes treatment goals, is accountable for revising these as treatment moves on, and, as well, for monitoring treatment outcome.

2

Beyond the physician–patient model: the value of a treatment team for dealing with clinical complexity

Think about "best practices" (Bogan & English, 1994). A reassuring phrase, to be sure. Best practice guidelines are ideally "evidence based" and derived from research, the highest standard of which involve randomized controlled trials. The product is relatively precise, leading to one or more decision trees (algorithms) with steps outlined for going from one point to another clinically.

It is important to be aware, however, that these guidelines are formulated on the basis of group data from studies conducted under controlled circumstances. Adjustments are frequently necessary when applying them to individual cases. For example, how does one reconcile these well-conceived sequences with the ever-present problem of a patient who refuses a critical procedure, who stops taking his or her medication, or who misses appointments? What about the patient who simply doesn't like your style or decisions and abruptly decides to switch physicians? And, then, of course, there are those for whom one or more of these protocols just don't work. Said in another way, in clinical work the vicissitudes of commitment resulting from the patient's and physician's individual needs and subjective responses are always present, potentially confounding the treatment situation.

We are not intending to be pessimistic. Just realistic. In this book we take on the issue of accountability in clinical practice; how the physician can tighten his or her work and use measures that include collaboration with others to come up with the desired results. In spite of the ubiquitous approximations incorporated into them, statistical analyses are helpful for establishing the efficacy of clinical proced-ures. We also have our careful reading of the literature to keep us on track. Our intention in this book is to organize these contributions to clinical practice into a coherent approach. More centrally, however, and to this end, in Chapter 1 we reviewed the technical enhancements to the clinical process we call "truing measures." Repeating our definition, "*truing*" in clinical practice refers to techniques through which a physician can improve and track the accuracy of his or her work.

As mentioned in Chapter 1, "truing" is one application of the principle of "successive approximations," a method for sequentially improving the precision of a series of observations or decisions by repeated reference to one or more related known quantities; in our case clinical data.[1] Said differently, a truing sequence consists of: incremental steps involving trial, error, and correction, used in arriving at an increasingly precise determination about the validity of a clinical action or procedure.

Moving beyond the truing measures listed in Chapter 1 for improving precision in a practitioner's individual work with a patient, we find ourselves in the territory of the treatment team. These are the people – professional, patient, and family members as potential collaborators – who are centrally implicated in the treatment of complex cases. The individual practitioner and the treatment team are two of the main platforms from which treatment is conducted. This book is organized around these foci, with the objective of progressively elaborating ways the physician working in each context can achieve desired results and measure progress.

The physician and the patient: dyadic versus team-based treatment

Most people think about the relationship between the physician and patient as essentially comprised of two people. You are the patient's primary physician. He or she comes to you with a list of problems. These are accorded priorities, either explicitly or implicitly. The ranking may be done more or less collaboratively, but the physician member of the pair ultimately has the responsibility of ordering and directing the work.

Truing comes in as the physician and patient attempt to find their way clinically. Among other responsibilities, it is incumbent on the physician to both facilitate and monitor progress, making sure the work is in line with outcome measures set toward the beginning of the treatment (Epstein, 1983; Cohen, 1988; Sturm *et al.*, 1999; Groopman, 2007; Bohmer & Lee, 2009; Knaup *et al.*, 2009).

Moving back to the treatment team, how many clinical situations do you know of that actually consist of only two influential people? Apart from an assortment of physicians, there are often, at minimum, several other professionals, including allied healthcare workers and specialists who at times make up the balance of the team. Most commonly, there is also a spouse, and sometimes children and other relatives, who may provide input for the team and communicate with appropriate team members. At times, there are also people with authority from the patient's employment or cultural world. Heading up

---

[1] A related concept familiar in industry and applied to healthcare administration is "continuous quality improvement."

this entire process is a team coordinator who, according to our model for work with the complex cases, is an MPCP.

As mentioned in Chapter 1, when treatment is constituted according to our team-based, collaborative model, truing occurs on two levels. (1) The first level (Level 1) is specific to the specialization of each of the physicians and other healthcare providers associated with the treatment team. This, the "micro" level, is comprised of these professionals in an assortment of dyadic encounters with patients. (2) The second, the "macro" level (Level 2), centers around the MPCP, who coordinates the treatment and oversees the treatment team. "Level 1" ("micro"), then, is made up of direct service providers. "Level 2" ("macro") encompasses the MPCP's coordinating, goal setting, and monitoring activities.

The treatment team, its complexities

We have not yet fully delineated the MPCP's contribution to the treatment process. First, the potential negatives. One cannot simply assume that a team structure will necessarily result in better outcomes than a dyadic one. The greater the number of people on the treatment team the more room there is for differences of opinion. Furthermore, physicians may work at cross purposes to each other, as they did in Keith's case, described below. Communication among team members may be hard to arrange and maintain. The patient may be "lost" in a multi-person operation, the focus on the patient's welfare disappearing in its busyness.

But, as noted above, thinking about most treatments as plainly dyadic is usually an over-simplification. Treatment of complex patients almost always involves the services and input of several people working coordinately. It stands to reason, then, that for "clinically and operationally complex" cases a thought-fully constituted and maintained treatment team is likely to deliver systemic medical and psychiatric services that are more focused and sophisticated than can be expected in either a two-person treatment situation or a loosely consti-tuted treatment effort involving more than one provider (Gittell *et al.*, 2000; Bodenheimer, 2007; Gittell *et al.*, 2008; Bohmer & Lee, 2009; Gittell, 2009; Nutting *et al.*, 2009; Hinami *et al.*, 2010).

Returning to the MPCP-led model, teams need rules, enforcers for these rules, and people who can provide organization. Even more to the point, whoever organizes and coordinates a treatment team needs to understand the technical issues governing outcome. Included, is setting and following outcome measures and keeping all team members accountable for their contribution not only to the team but, more centrally, to the patient. Throughout the book we will have a great deal more to say about the MPCP concept and its implementation. However, since this book is essentially about patients and their narratives, it is time to bring one in. Here is part one of Keith's story. The rest will be told in Chapter 6.

Keith

A patient with a history of polycythemia vera for almost 20 years, Keith fearlessly bucked his disease. He was a nearly "perfect" patient, rarely questioning his physician's orders. He had required monthly phlebotomies for several years, and managed admirably with a number of complications of polycythemia vera including peptic ulcer disease, gouty arthritis, and erythromelalgia (burning pain affecting his feet and hands). Keith was also loyal, and, as we will illustrate later, perhaps at times too loyal.

Keith's primary care physician, Dr. R., was indeed meticulous. His workups were thorough, his treatments absolutely up to date. From a two-person, physician–patient treatment model involving medical treatment alone, he was as "perfect" as a physician as Keith was as a patient. As you can imagine, Keith liked Dr. R, believing Dr. R. cared deeply for him and would always do what was medically best for him.

All well and good. But, there were also irregularities. The first was the "dual relationship" Dr. R. maintained with Keith (Lazarus & Zur, 2002; Zur, 2011). Keith was both patient and friend to Dr. R. You already know about the patient side. As friends, Keith and Dr. R. spent hours together on the golf links, and here is where problems came in.

Medically "perfect" as he was, Dr. R. neglected and distorted certain standard truing provisions. These fell into two categories. The first had to do with outcome measures. In setting these, Dr. R. was technically sophisticated as far as medical issues were concerned. But, he was far from the mark in his understanding of, and even interest in, Keith's wishes.

Complicating things even further, however, was that Keith's desires were in conflict with those of his daughters. Keith wanted to maintain his dignity during the terminal phase of his illnesses. He was not particularly afraid of dying. But, he was worried about losing self-respect as his disease progressed and its complications mounted. In competition with Keith's wishes, his daughters were afraid of losing their father and wanted his life prolonged at all costs. And, oh yes, there was Keith's wife. She was an accomplished, sensible woman who was the most realistic member of the group. You now have before you the informal treatment "team" as it existed at that point.

Notice there are no additional physicians involved yet, so the "team" consisted of Keith, family members who were divided among themselves about Keith's care, and Keith's primary physician, Dr. R. The pressing question at that point was how to set outcome measures and who should determine them? Whose wishes should prevail? According to conventional wisdom, clearly Keith, while competent, should have his desires in the forefront. Unfortunately, however, as skilled as Dr. R. was with medical matters, that level of clinical consideration seemed to elude him.

The second truing principle Dr. R. neglected was the detachment required for exercising reasonable objectivity. Dr. R. was first and foremost a dedicated researcher whose area of investigation was myeloproliferative disorders. Keith, we infer, was relevant to him in more ways than one. No doubt Dr. R. had a strong medical conscience and, as a friend of sorts, cared personally for Keith. But there was something more at issue. Dr. R. was intensely, scientifically, curious about certain biological aspects of Keith's disease, and perhaps a bit overly enthusiastic about the treatments he was rendering. In brief, all else aside, there are indications that Keith was a scientifically fascinating project for Dr. R. Detachment, then, was missing on two fronts: the personal and the scientific.

There was also a third deficiency. Dr. R. proved to be uninterested in medical points of view other than his own. As far as we know Dr. R. rarely, if ever, consulted with other physicians as difficulties arose in this case. We are referring both to his obvious ignoring of Keith's and Keith's family's personal needs and preferences, as well his neglecting the disabling impact on Keith of his deteriorating condition. In fact, the more appropriate consultations with other physicians, especially those involving psychiatric matters, became, the more resistant Dr. R. seemed to become about using them.

You can probably see where we are leading. This case description is intended to serve as a further introduction to the topic of truing measures that are useful in guiding clinical work, and the value of a treatment team with a single coordinating physician, an MPCP, with leadership responsibility for "clinically and operationally complex" cases. Keith's situation became "operationally complex" as more people with conflicting viewpoints were involved in his case, and, as you will see in following chapters, it also evolved to become "diagnostically complex" as his illness progressed.

This book

The single, abiding question we attempt to address throughout this book is how a physician can be reasonably assured of getting the best results, especially in complex cases that challenge his or her skills. The "medical model" involves the following three-part sequence.[2] (1) Beginning with the patient's presenting problems, (2) the physician gets the data necessary for confirmation or revision of the prevailing hypotheses about the nature and etiology of the patient's problems. (3) When the physician's understanding is reasonably reliable, he or she moves toward the interventions that are most likely to be effective.

---

[2] The "medical model" has been the traditional approach to the diagnosis and treatment of illness as practiced by physicians in the Western world at least since the time of Koch and Pasteur. The physician focuses on the defect, or dysfunction, within the patient, using a problem-solving approach. The medical history, physical examination, and diagnostic tests provide the basis for the identification and treatment of a specific illness. The medical model is thus focused on the physical and biologic aspects of specific diseases and conditions. (*Mosby's Medical Dictionary*, 8th edition. © 2009, Elsevier.)

Much of this book is about this sequence, identifying a methodology that allows us to confirm or reject hypotheses about the patient's condition and choose the best ways to treat it. We place emphasis on the organizing and coordinating function required in complex clinical situations, and will go to great lengths to elaborate the role of the physician who provides that function, the medical–psychiatric coordinating physician (MPCP).

Effective clinical work requires the constant infusion of intuition, clinical judgment, strategic thinking, and collaboration with the patient, other physicians, and additional healthcare professionals. Chapters that follow will be devoted to these topics. But, the focal point for all these chapters remains simply that of achieving the best possible outcomes: how to arrive at them, how to know they are optimal, how to be sure they are enduring, and who should oversee this process.

When customary truing practices are neglected: examples of omitted truing

Dr. R. was always clear about Keith's major complaints, at least the medical ones. He did his best to understand Keith's polycythemia vera. It was in acknowledging the progressive operational complexity of Keith's situation and honoring Keith's wishes where Dr. R. failed.

Compare Keith's situation to Nel, who we offer as representing a "clinically complex" case with prominent psychiatric elements and in which standard truing measures were also omitted. In this instance the patient came for treatment at her husband's insistence. Her husband was "alarmed" because of "her frequent angry outbursts." These had been evident for about a year, and as a result she allegedly was "alienating friends and family members." According to him she also had a reputation for being insensitive, putting people off with "her often too-direct, disparaging judgments." Her husband characterized her behavior as "ADHD-like" and insisted she needed "anger management counseling, medication, and psychotherapy." He paid almost no attention to the fact that these episodes came in bursts and had on occasion been described by others as "seizure-like." There were other signs suggesting possible neurological involvement, but these were not taken into account until much later. At first, Nel concurred with her husband's opinions and reported that she too was alarmed. She was starting to believe her husband's allegations about her "misbehavior," and was concerned that the marriage could fail if she "didn't cooperate in dealing with her problems immediately."

Enter Dr. E., an experienced psychiatrist who specialized in work with couples and families. The encounter was initiated by Nel's husband, who called him asking for "couples' treatment." In response, without speaking to Nel, her previous psychiatrist, or undertaking any other assessments, Dr. E. scheduled two meetings for the couple. As might be expected from the way the initial contact was made and handled, it was the husband's allegations about her condition that were most persuasive to Dr. E.

Dr. E. acted fast. His initial measures, based on the first two conjoint meetings and a self-assessment screening for ADHD (Attention-Deficit/Hyperactivity Disorder), included a trial of amphetamine plus dextroamphetamine to address Nel's suspected ADHD, the recommendation of cognitive behavioral therapy for anger management, and "couples' treatment" with himself for Nel and her husband. In taking this path Dr. E. was clearly bypassing the potential neurological aspects of the case and responding primarily to the psychiatric and social issues as he understood them.

As a parallel to this case, consider another clinical situation involving a debilitating upper respiratory condition that has lingered for six months and has been unresponsive to a standard antibiotic treatment. Imagine the involved physician concluding, before getting any further studies, that the next step in the management of the case should be a different antibiotic or antiviral regimen. There is no attempt to take more history, do repeat medical examinations, initiate consultations with other physicians, and no consideration of obtaining additional laboratory tests or diagnostic imaging studies. Hard to picture, isn't it? The problems with the way these two cases, Nel's and this one, were handled is obvious. An adequately dedicated application of the medical model, the primary physician following reasonable clinical and laboratory or psychometric assessment sequences, has been omitted in both situations. Again, proper diagnostic and management considerations in psychiatry and systemic medicine align.

And, the outcomes? You already must have an impression of what happened to Keith as a result of Dr. R.'s insistence on doing things in his own way without additional input. In a general sense Nel's fate was similar. Over the next few months Nel's "rage episodes" worsened, and signs clearly suggestive of a neurological condition, including problems with balance and coordination, became progressively evident. Dr. E. had acted too quickly in accepting Nel's husband's allegations and failing to obtain the additional information necessary to make a thorough assessment of the situation. In effect, he was bypassing the diagnostic complexity of the case. A possible neurological etiology for Nel's symptoms had not been seriously enough considered; nor had the distortion in case management that might result from complicity between himself and Nel's husband. Perhaps, though, this misconceived intervention had a paradoxical silver lining for Nel. In the end, the unacknowledged alliance between Dr. E. and Nel's husband became so blatant that even Nel began to "get it." This was the point at which Nel began to talk about divorce.

Keith's experience with Dr. R. provides a good example of the limited attention that may unwittingly be given to the full range of a patient's needs by an overly-busy or preoccupied PCP; especially when that physician is working in relative isolation. In Keith's case there was little consideration given to his personal requirements, including his devotion to his family and theirs to him. It was also important that Dr. R. understand Keith's wife's and adult children's attitudes about his end-stage disease and its treatment. For Nel, a more rigorous stance about evaluation, approaching it more methodically, could probably have saved her from a misguided treatment effort, the underestimation of a neurological contribution to her condition, and attendant marital disruption.

The MPCP

Move to the requirements for functioning as an MPCP. Required is enough in-depth understanding of individual psychology to grasp the more elusive aspects of a patient's emotional life and how these may influence the course of treatment. Needed for that role is familiarity with family and social systems, including knowledge of how to deal with the knotty administrative and psychological challenges of coordinating a treatment team. There are numerous other subject areas where this kind of experience can be helpful. For example, as a physician you may not know much more than the basics about less-central but related clinical areas such as child development and the ways a child may influence the family and, in turn, upset its homeostatic balance. Also, you may not have much experience in working with institutions and agencies apart from hospitals.

In addition to broad clinical knowledge and competence, the MPCP must relate credibly to the others involved in the patient's care, including other physicians and healthcare professionals. The MPCP also needs to be able to set and modify treatment goals as well as understand how to ascertain that required progress is occurring. Familiarity with medical statistics and clinical evaluation techniques is helpful here. Add, the requirement that the MPCP comprehend cultural issues as they influence the patient's life and expectations.

Note, the above list contains psychological and social considerations that are often undervalued in primary care practice, especially when systemic medical issues are pressing. Nonetheless, in one way or another, the subject areas listed all have to do with the ways a patient understands or reacts to illness, as well as cooperates with treatment. They also touch on the MPCP's role in that process. In our experience in work with "clinically complex" cases, psychosocial considerations are often on equal footing with those that are clearly systemic medical and psychiatric.

Not yet discussed is the place of medical training in preparing for MPCP work, its clinical, diagnostic, and operational complexity. Clearly, when complex cases have significant psychiatric co-morbidity, that is co-morbidity with prominent psychiatric components, it is a great advantage and often necessary for the MPCP to be a psychiatrist. Training to be an MPCP will be discussed in Chapter 11. Many of the fundamental skill sets required to become an MPCP can be gained through psychiatric residencies as well as the proper selection of fellowships. However, additional training in work with complicated medical and social systems, including treatment teams, is clearly advantageous for assuming that role.

The complexities of the MPCP's job: Nel continued

Return to Nel and her husband. Put yourself into the mind of a psychiatrist called in to help; this time not Dr. E. but instead an MPCP.

Let's break the problem confronting this physician into its components. First, his or her initial hypotheses about how to structure the evaluation at the point of referral.

(1) In this case the referral comes from the patient's husband. This would be a warning sign for a psychiatrist who is working from a family systems perspective. Most likely that psychiatrist's first thought is that the contact should have come from the patient herself. Consequently, the workup would probably begin with the patient. Clinical criteria would then be used to decide if and how to incorporate her husband.

(2) The initial screening reveals that, in addition to rage episodes, Nel had recently complained about "absence spells," intermittent loss of balance and some problems with coordination for a period of at least a year, and trouble staying awake during the daytime. No one as yet had suggested that she see a neurologist, but given this set of symptoms that certainly would make sense.

(3) If the allegation of episodes of anger and rage is accurate, and if, as a result of a negative electro encephalogram (EEG) and neurological workup, these behaviors appear not to be manifestations of partial complex seizures (psychomotor epilepsy), more extensive medical, neurological, and psychiatric workups, including psychometric assessment, would be in order.

So far, however, this approach is mainly a conception in the psychiatrist's mind, since she or he barely has been able to gather background data from Nel and her husband. This is the point for the psychiatrist to begin to think about team creation. As the treatment begins to take shape, the psychiatrist, in collaboration with the patient, will need to progressively fix on initial treatment goals. As you well know from your own experience as a physician, this is the way it goes clinically. You start with a series of informal hypotheses, you progressively gather the information necessary to refine and revise these, and you end up with a set of new hypotheses which allow you to formulate an initial treatment strategy.

Returning to the actual case, additional, complicating, psychological and interpersonal issues became evident at this point. A new psychiatrist with a specialization in neurology, who had at first been called in as a consultant, eventually moved to the position of MPCP and needed to deal with these. At the point of the second psychiatrist's initial involvement, Nel's husband still continued to believe that Dr. E. "walked on water" and that he had "definitively" diagnosed Nel's problem. The husband considered the new psychiatrist "incompetent," since he didn't automatically accept the view that Nel was the one who was psychologically troubled and that her difficulties were the crux of the clinical problem. Given Dr. E.'s remaining influence, even at this point both Nel and her husband were still skeptical about the need for an extensive neurological workup.

Illustrated here is the complicated diagnostic and management role of the MPCP. When he finally moved to the role of MPCP, the new psychiatrist's charge became working with Nel and her husband to make sure missing diagnostic information was obtained, acted upon, and that the couple's differences were addressed. It was also important for him to confirm that Nel understood and was in agreement with new diagnostic findings, which at this point included "partial complex seizures," and for him to organize all treatment participants, including Nel's PCP, into a formal, cooperating treatment team.

So there is no mystery, the marriage did not survive. The divorce occurred three years later.

Returning to Keith, you already know how messy that situation was almost from the beginning. Keith's main physician, Dr. R., had no real use for Keith's family's or his wife's opinion. The more these people asserted themselves, the more difficult it became to collaborate with him. Keith's personal needs, of course, went entirely unheeded. Think of how fortunate Keith would have been if his primary care from the start had been placed in the hands of a physician with training and interest in both systemic medicine and psychiatry, who was willing to work with the complex psychosocial situation that came to characterize the case, and was willing to bring in appropriate specialists.

Leadership and the MPCP

We have been emphasizing the organizing function of the MPCP, the interface of that person's responsibility for the patient and his or her work with other involved professionals. We need to add that among the team members there is always a PCP who provides the balance of the systemic medical treatment when the MPCP is not current in *both* psychiatry and systemic medicine. Active collaboration between the MPCP and PCP is, of course, particularly critical for the treatment team to function optimally.

So far, however, we have said relatively little about the *direct* benefits to the treatment of the MPCP's unique role. The MPCP, while team leader, generally also assumes some direct treatment functions such a prescribing medication, performing psychiatric and, at times, systemic medical workups, or doing individual and/or family psychotherapy. In part because of these combined responsibilities, we actually understand the MPCP to be treating the "pathology," the dysfunctions, afflicting the patient's medical and psychosocial system as a unit. We will provide examples of this clinical role throughout the book. In this capacity the MPCP provides organization, including a sense of purpose, future, and motivation for the overall treatment process. To do this work he or she needs to understand the psychology of all team members, including that of the patient, and be skilled at formulating strategies that capture the patient's, and, in many cases, the family's interest and commitment. Furthermore, when working with clinically and operationally complex cases, there are generally crises that can subvert the treatment. While critical for maintenance of the case, the MPCP's competent management of these incidents also serves the important purpose of reinforcing team members' confidence in the overall treatment effort.

This list is just a start. We will say a good deal more about the MPCP in future chapters.

Steps along the way

We now return to clinical practice proper and begin our odyssey from the procedures that aid in delivering the most reliable care, truing measures, to the final elaboration of our fully integrated treatment model for working with diagnostically and operationally complex cases.

Returning to our truing measures, there is one category which stands out as particularly useful for providing reliable help in clinical situations. Laboratory tests and diagnostic imaging studies in the field of systemic medicine qualify for this designation, as do psychometric assessments in psychiatry. In Chapter 3 we discuss how these procedures fit into our diagnostic and treatment sequence.

3

Sorting out clinical complexity: medical and psychometric testing

No contemporary subject in medicine has received more attention than empirical verification for treatment decisions, formalized as "evidence-based treatments" (EBTs), "evidence-based medicine" (EBM), and "empirically supported treatments" (ESTs)[1] (Chambless & Hollon, 1998; Woolf & George, 2000; Beutler, 2009; Straus et al., 2010). In recent years there has been a push to ground treatments with data, ideally data derived from randomized assignment of patients to specified treatment conditions. The result: treatment manuals with step-by-step intervention instructions, frequently in the form of algorithms.

OK, so who is right in the "science versus sentiment" controversy (Frank & Frank, 1991; Matthews, 1997; Wampold, 2001; Norcross, 2002; Fox, 2008; Gelso, 2009)? The authors of this book are thoroughly encouraged by the trend toward validating treatments by measurable outcomes. And, yet, we are also concerned by pressures to rely too excessively on evidence-based treatment protocols with the relative devaluing of what we label "experience-based clinical judgment" (EBCJ).

In Chapters 4 and 5 we show that the complexity of clinical work with patients goes well beyond the reductionistic syndrome and symptom-oriented approach of manualized treatment protocols. Imagine that you are a patient going to an internist who "does it strictly by the book" and fails to take the patient's personal experience of illness into account. Say your presenting complaint is "shortness of breath." You are aware of the potential relationship of recent onset breathing difficulties with cardiac disease. However, you are 76 years old and heart disease isn't all that concerns you. A few well-placed questions from the internist would have revealed that you've recently been preoccupied by a sense of dread that you could stop breathing in the middle of the night. At those times your imagination goes wild. When these thoughts occur, you become obsessed with trying to catch

---

[1] While often used synonymously, the term "empirically based" or "empirically supported" is more widely associated with psychology and the applied behavioral sciences, and "evidence based" is more generally used in systemic medicine and psychiatry.

your breath, and, of course, your anxiety leads to hyperventilation in a vicious cycle. The algorithm your internist uses, however, is only minimally pertinent for your situation. It emphasizes cardiac and pulmonary explanations for your symptoms and the next steps on the decision tree are all in the systemic medical realm.

So, where does that leave us as physicians? The development of evidence-based medicine is here to stay and that's a good thing. But since, with evidence-based approaches, we run the risk of losing the broader, patient-centered context, we need to retain an experiential, judgment-based perspective as well.

There is an inherent tension between these two large trends. Evidence-based medicine (Straus *et al.*, 2010) seeks to standardize treatment along group norms, while "patient-centered treatment" (Institute of Medicine of the National Academies, 2001; Shaller, 2007) focuses on the needs of the particular patient. In our MPCP model, we attempt to reconcile these points of view. There is clearly use for an EBM-type approach when working with "diagnostically complex" cases; for example, patients with chronic or otherwise treatment-intensive systemic illness and psychiatric co-morbidity. Once the patient is so defined, however, the MPCP-led model of care takes over and provides a more patient-centered, personalized, approach to the needs of the patient, always referring to EBM methods when clinically appropriate (Epstein, 1983).

Be reassured, though. There's more to this picture. We don't have to be stuck with only those two choices – evidence-based treatments or clinical judgment. We do have markers that will allow us to follow a patient's course with considerable precision. These guides, the range of truing methods available to us, can enable us to stay on track or modify our direction if we are not. Of the truing measures we have described so far, typically, the most powerful one is testing, e.g. laboratory and diagnostic imaging in systemic medicine, and neuropsychological and personality (psychometric) assessments in psychiatry. Recall, however, that this is a forced dichotomy, since psychometric instruments, particularly brief and practical ones, are increasingly used in systemic medicine, and laboratory and diagnostic imaging have become even more crucial in psychiatric practice.

Ambiguity in clinical testing

However, all clinical testing has its ambiguities and sources of imprecision. Laboratory and diagnostic imaging assessments are no exception (Cheek, 1982; Hummel, 1999). In a sophisticated and extensive review of the validity of both systemic-medical and psychological assessments, Meyer *et al.* (2001) and Meyer (2003) found the two to be roughly comparable in accuracy. It is probably worth taking a moment to consider this finding. Radiological reports and laboratory findings usually have to be interpreted before they are of any use. Similarly, psychometric tests are usually administered and interpreted by a psychologist. And, any time that professionals interpret data there will be differences of opinion. So, testing of any sort is never truly completely "objective."

Combine these sources of uncertainty with the chaotic experience of working with complex cases, and the importance of incorporating reliable truing activities into clinical work becomes especially evident. The four case examples that follow illustrate both "diagnostic complexity" and "operational complexity" (refer to Chapter 1 for definitions of these terms). In keeping with its definition, the "operational complexity" is associated with the interactions among the multiple physicians and healthcare professionals who became involved in the care of these patients. Absent in each of the following cases was a formal treatment team and case coordinator.

Assessment in systemic medicine: false positives and false negatives

Diane: a disturbing false positive

Fifty-three-year-old Diane was still dripping with sensuality. After all, that is how she had initially attracted her ex-husband, a wealthy attorney. For years following their divorce, because of concern for their two children, he continued to support her at a financially extravagant level. But time was running out. The children were in high school and termination of mandatory alimony had already occurred.

That's when she had the first episode of ataxia, followed in weeks by numbness in her right arm. She was astute enough to seize on multiple sclerosis as a diagnosis which could qualify her to have her support extended and eventually make her eligible for disability payments. It was also license to dump much of the responsibility for the children on her ex-husband, since she was "too sick" to care for them. Instead, she needed to shift her attention and begin her quixotic odyssey, moving from physician to physician, seeking those who would agree with her desired diagnosis and empathize with her plight. Multiple sclerosis was a good choice of disease for Diane, since apart from equivocal cerebrospinal fluid (CSF) findings, neuroimaging showing CNS plaques, non-specific irregularities in somatosensory evoked potentials, and biopsies demonstrating destruction of myelin sheaths of nerve fibers, there are no definitive clinical tests for it.

Remarkable in this case was Diane's ability to find physicians who came up with a diagnosis of multiple sclerosis. She attached herself to these physicians after seeing several who were quite clear that she did not have convincing clinical or laboratory evidence of that disease. At about that point she also turned to attorneys to argue for a continuation of her alimony support payments and, as might be predicted, had several suspicious episodes involving numbness, weakness, and ataxia that panicked her children and ex-husband, and clinched her case for financial support.

Dorothy

Dorothy had made her mark. She was a prominent, published professor of psychology at a prestigious university. And then she began to disappear. She grew weak, experienced fevers, and became depressed. What was this illness? How could it be happening to such a vital, dynamic individual? Did she have an occult cancer? Did she pick up a parasitic infection on her recent trip to Africa? Maybe this was one of those chronic, "slow viruses"? Thus began an exhaustive series of tests at university medical centers. But, nothing much showed up. The only positive findings were an increased erythrocyte sedimentation rate and antibodies to the Epstein–Barr virus: about as non-specific as any immunological findings could be.

Dorothy *knew* she had something "real," but progressively her physicians opted out. They were thoughtful and kind, but there was "nothing yet to treat." There were medications to try but all had major side effects, were expensive, and several were experimental and not covered by her health insurance plan. So, Dorothy decided to pass on them. All the while she was pleading, shrieking for someone to take her seriously, to not give up on her. Yet, that is exactly what they did. Physicians have more than their share of such patients. After several extensive workups and some difficulty with patient compliance, they hardly have enough time to wrestle with cases that continue not to make sense to them. That level of commitment becomes even more problematic if there is no obvious financial support for the proposed diagnostic procedures and treatments. The MPCP role, in contrast, is designed to avoid such eventualities. In part these incidents occur because, with fragmentation of care, there may not be any single physician who is designated to take responsibility for coordinating a patient's care and monitoring its outcome.

Dorothy faded from sight. The word was that she had "given up." Friends heard nothing from her for six months, when they suddenly received news of her death.

Flora

Flora's symptoms were like Dorothy's, with similar ambiguous laboratory results. But, she had a "reason" to be depressed. For years she had a fiefdom as the assistant headteacher at a wealthy private preparatory school. Her largesse and her unconditional availability endeared her to all except those who got close to her. To that small group of people she had come to seem self-righteous.

Born in the Republic of South Africa, Flora lived on the school campus. She had no other social life. She was divorced and had no children. In fact, her "ownership" of the students with whom she spent hour after hour could, on close inspection, seem a bit out of line, an illusion that these were in effect "her children." Flora seemed to thrive on the idea that she had a very special, maternal role in each of their lives.

Inevitably things changed. First, the headmaster began to see her as a nuisance. Then he attempted to cut back her duties. She retrenched, attempted to muster support from parents and teachers, and eventually hired an attorney, threatening to sue the school, alleging violation of her contract. At first she did not become overtly depressed, but she did become ill. Muscle pains, diagnosed eventually as fibromyalgia, complaints of fevers, and general debilitation came to dominate her life. As with Dorothy, physician appointments grew exponentially. Then, depression, isolation, and the development of a delusional belief that the deterioration of her authority with students was the product of a conspiracy involving administrators, teachers, and even students. In concert with these developments the school progressively, but unsuccessfully, tried to get rid of her.

At that point, the headmaster moved to a new school and a different one replaced him. The incoming headmaster was not as personally embroiled with Flora as the one who had left. It wasn't long, in fact, before the new headmaster settled Flora's legal claim, asked her leave, and hired another assistant headteacher to replace her. And, that is about where Flora's physical decline started in earnest.

Flora's grievances escalated and eventually took on a paranoid flavor. She almost stopped eating, isolated herself, and eventually required two psychiatric hospitalizations. Following her second hospitalization she returned to live with her siblings in the Republic of South Africa.

Joshua

A high-powered engineer, a partner in a small, high-tech startup company, Joshua claimed that he was eventually "misused" by his business partners. When his small, originally promising company was hit by a series of lawsuits about malfunctioning products, he stepped up to the plate, attempting to do his part to set things straight. The problem is that none of the others did the same. He hung in until the end, always the fall guy. And, of course, he grew resentful.

Married twice and divorced each time, Joshua was childless. One day, his first wife, whom he "loved" and admired, told him that she was a lesbian. Sadly, a few years later, she died from suicide. Joshua's dreams of reconciliation went up in smoke. He married again, but that marriage was ill-fated because the two were of different ethnicities, he American from the Midwest and she Indian from a traditional family. He did his best to make himself acceptable to her parents, but apparently that was not enough to satisfy them and the marriage failed. What did he have left? A younger sister and nephew, both of whom he loved, a few friends, and an idealized past in the engineering and business worlds. To some extent even this picture was threatened by his sister's progressive dementia.

Joshua's early history was contributory. The product of a missionary family, he rarely lived in one location for more than a few years. These moves required that as a child he change schools often. His mother had an affair while the family was in Africa. A child resulted, instigating a crisis that nearly destroyed the family. This instability was too much for the patient's father who became morbidly depressed and eventually lapsed into psychosis. Joshua took care of him until his early twenties.

After the high-tech business broke up, Joshua was left to deal with lawyers. Devastated, too exhausted to cope, he filed for disability and withdrew socially.

And, it got worse. He progressively isolated himself and could not get up the energy to return to work. A life washed up.

It was about this time that Joshua caught on to the diagnosis of Chronic Fatigue Syndrome. His logical, unemotional demeanor couldn't incorporate a primarily psychiatric diagnosis, so he was unwilling, perhaps unable, to consider "depression" as the medical cause of his impaired function. The psychiatrist he consulted could see it clearly, but Joshua could not. Consequently he was reluctant to enter psychotherapy, and simply relied on self-help books to find his way. Medication was offered but he declined to take it. Years later, in spite of moderate improvement in his mood, he still was loath to consider depression as at least a partial explanation for his physical symptoms. Supporting his claim of systemic physical illness, there also were some non-specific systemic medical findings. His erythrocyte sedimentation rate (ESR) was intermittently elevated, along with his Epstein–Barr virus (EBV) antibody and anti-nuclear antibody (ANA) titers. Additionally, above and beyond debilitating fatigue, he occasionally experienced low-grade fevers.

Thirteen years later, Joshua still was relatively isolated. He had a disabled sister and niece, one cousin with whom he regularly spent time, a few old friends, and took a bit more interest in the world. He mainly occupied himself by developing an esoteric electronic device. Of note, however, he was too frightened to attempt to patent and market this invention. He earned some money doing computer work for a friend. As always, he remained efficient and meticulous. However, even minimal physical activity quickly left him "exhausted," and he limited his social and vocational commitments accordingly.

Joshua's visits to physician after physician earned him the diagnosis, Chronic Fatigue Syndrome. With medical support for this diagnosis, he prevailed with his insurance carrier and received extended disability payments.

Summing up

The four patients just described are not particularly unusual in primary care practices. Patients with similar diffuse or unsubstantiated complaints are encountered by PCPs all the time. They may get referred to psychiatrists, their PCPs certain their illnesses are basically psychiatric. The patients are convinced they have a systemic disease, often a progressive one. They may be overtly manipulative like Diane, but often they are not. They are just looking for a unifying systemic diagnosis, at times validation that they have one, and for some kind of treatment for their disorder. In a case like Diane's, the physicians they ultimately find may validate the patient's claim. History and physical examination may equivocally support it, and medical tests are ambiguous enough to convince them that the patient may be right. Also, these physicians are aware that many diseases present first with non-specific symptoms such as weight loss, low-grade fevers, and myalgias. Occult cancers, for example, may start out that way. It is only later that a true diagnosis can be made.

Comprehensive personality and neuropsychological (psychometric) assessment

The terms "psychological assessment" and "psychometric assessment" are synonymous, and "personality assessment" and "neuropsychological assessment" are subcategories of both.[2] Psychometric assessment comes in at least three varieties.

(1) Relatively brief, self-report and self-assessment as well as clinician assisted batteries: Examples include the SCL-90 (the Symptom Check List – 90) (Derogatis, 2000), and the Beck and Hamilton Depression and Anxiety scales (Hamilton, 1960; Beck *et al.*, 1996).

(2) Test batteries for the purpose of "personality assessment:" among these are the MMPI-2 (Minnesota Multiphasic Psychological Inventory) (Ben-Porath & Tellegen, 2008), and unstructured "performance-based tests" (traditionally called "projective tests") that probe the patient's inner world, and include the Thematic Apperception Test (TAT) (Murray, 1943) and the Rorschach "inkblot test" (Rorschach, 1921).

(3) Comprehensive test battery groupings, each group constituting a neuropsychological assessment: in this book we also refer to this level of assessment as "comprehensive psychometric assessment."

Assessment in psychiatry and psychology hold the same promise as laboratory and diagnostic imaging in systemic medicine and are fraught with similar sources of imprecision. In addition to test imprecision, there is the subjectivity introduced by both the examiner and the psychologist who interprets the results.

Think of a testing protocol that is made up of 20 or so individual tests. This is the magnitude of a comprehensive neuropsychological test battery consisting of "localizing" measures of CNS dysfunction, and, as well, frequently, of personality assessment protocols. The objective of this kind of assessment is to distinguish cortically based problems such as those that involve executive functions, memory, attention, and cognition, from those like depression that are more specifically associated with subcortical structures. This distinction is not absolute, as some cortical lesions such as stroke are associated with depression, while illnesses with a predominantly subcortical location, such as Parkinson's disease, are associated with cognitive impairment. Our experience with Victor, age 25,

---

[2] As we discuss psychological assessment in psychiatry we need to be clear about definitions. As commonly employed, the labels "psychometric assessment" and "psychological assessment" are synonymous. The proper use of the term "psychometric assessment," however, in contrast to "psychological assessment," places emphasis on measurement rather than on the description of individual personality traits and dysfunctions. As well, the field of psychometrics is especially concerned with the structure and characteristics of assessment protocols. Nonetheless, "psychometric" is the more commonly employed term in medicine and as such will be used most frequently in this book when we refer to either psychological (personality) or neuropsychological assessment.

should serve as an illustration of the value of this variety of testing when confronted with a case involving "diagnostic complexity."

Victor: a diagnostic challenge

Victor's irritability appeared to be a manifestation of depression. He also had sustained a serious head injury when he was four years of age, leaving him unconscious for 14 hours. There were no obvious neurological sequelae from that episode. He had been abandoned by his father at age six, and he, his sister, and his mother lived close to poverty from that point. Throughout his early development he suffered from asthma and frequent upper respiratory illnesses, causing him to miss school for weeks on end. Multiple physicians had been involved in his care, each ultimately seeking psychiatric consultation.

Psychometric assessment at ages 8 and again at 15 focused on anxiety, related to fears of abandonment complicating an already consolidating "depressive core." Victor pessimistically saw everything as "black." He stopped trying to perform at school from an early point and failed to complete projects including those he claimed to like. He was generally devoid of emotion and for the most part avoided people.

Depression!

Or was it?

Luckily for Victor, his mother remarried when he was 16, and with the reestablishment of financial stability she and his stepfather decided that it might be useful to have Victor tested again, this time by a neuropsychologist to assess his associated attentional and learning, as well as emotional, problems.

And, indeed it was. The assessment had a "eureka" effect. In contrast to the previous personality assessment and the treating psychiatrist's clinical impression, neither depression nor anxiety dominated the test findings, although both were part of the clinical picture. Victor's testing also confirmed an already suspected attention deficit disorder, making it hard for him to remain interested in any task for very long, and discouraging him from trying in school. He was "deceptively smart," his verbal precocity influencing everyone to expect big things from him.

But, what about his irritability? Victor would flare up at odd times in response to seemingly benign provocations. How to explain these? Could they bear any relationship to his early head injury? Here is where the neuropsychological assessment had its greatest yield. Although suspected, the assessment did not reveal a significant learning disorder. Not clinically anticipated, however, but clear from the assessment, Victor was now showing indications of *Bipolar Disorder*, providing a more convincing explanation of his frequent, extreme mood shifts.

And the implications. Without this new information the psychiatrist might have continued to treat Victor with an antidepressant, running the risk of triggering an episode of mania. He also might not have searched again through Victor's family history and discovered the well-kept secrets that his father's mother had committed suicide after a lifetime of episodic but severe bouts of depression, and that each of his father's three brothers had substance abuse disorders.

Personality and neuropsychological assessment unlock two cases

Now to Mary and Margie and how psychological assessment made it possible to unravel their deceptions and the misconceptions surrounding their physical and psychological complaints. Note that in the following clinical descriptions the "I" is SAF, involved as the psychiatrist in both cases.

Mary: addiction masked as depression

After a long telephone conversation with her mother and stepfather, as well as another with her biological father, who lived in a different state, I met twice with Mary, age 22. In the first meeting, she was cooperative and articulate. To me she seemed remarkably forthcoming. She cited difficulty concentrating and a litany of alleged medical conditions to explain school failures that necessitated moves from one school to another beginning in the ninth grade. Included in her list of ailments were frequent episodes of abdominal pain, a condition she and her parents described as related to obscure ailments affecting her "liver and gall bladder" and "irritable bowel syndrome." In college she constantly struggled to focus and stay interested, but she was reportedly frequently preoccupied by her physical discomfort. Over years, she had seen multiple physicians for the purpose of diagnosing and treating her elusive symptoms.

In our first meeting, though, Mary was clear and cogent. However, the second interview was bewildering. Mary's thinking during that session seemed so tangential that I found myself considering some kind of CNS derangement or even a thought disorder as an explanation. The same pattern of inconsistency repeated itself through the third and fourth meetings. These sessions with Mary were flanked by meetings with her mother and stepfather, and phone calls with her biological father, for the purpose of gathering history, making sense of my clinical observations, and formulating a plan for an extended evaluation. I spoke with several of Mary's past and present physicians as well, but all were as confused as I was about Mary. The clinical picture remained unclear, framed by Mary's disarmingly cooperative manner in the midst of her fluctuating display of good and poor judgment, as well as alternating insightfulness about her personal instability and obtuseness about its possible causes.

Six weeks later, Mary again visited California from her home in a different state, this time for comprehensive psychometric assessment with a psychologist and several more meetings with me. During the intervening period I spoke with Mary on the telephone several times a week. While I also had telephone conversations with both her stepfather and mother, the main support for our work came from her stepfather. Mary's stepfather made the initial contact, insisted Mary keep her appointments, and pushed Mary's mother to see Mary's problems as urgent. He also progressively described his unrequited struggle to find a comfortable place for himself in this blended family; one where his concern for

Mary as well as his own needs could be heard and taken seriously. It was his tireless efforts, his willingness to join with me, that most powerfully supported my work with Mary and then redirected me to his wife's parenting failures and serious deficiencies in the marriage. However, at the point of these initial meetings, all I really knew was that Mary's unending medical complaints, school failures, and seeming irresponsibility had created havoc in her life and had her mother and stepfather greatly concerned.

At this point in the workup we turned to psychometric assessment[3] for clarification. In Mary's case, the results of this testing were eye-opening and focused our attention away from her medical complaints. According to the testing, Mary was experiencing substantial levels of stress and was so thoroughly dissociated from her feelings that she lacked the personal resources to find resolution. Most pointedly, the testing also exposed the fact that street drugs and alcohol were the only method she knew for finding relief, once her other attempts to manage her dilemma were exhausted. Mary had successfully hidden that fact from everyone.

In short, Mary was at the end of her rope emotionally, suffused with anxiety, and had no way out. To cope, she had seized on substances as the most reliable means of relief. Using these, Mary had become "slippery": clever enough to conceal her now exposed addiction to alcohol and barbiturates from everyone, including her parents. Her somatic symptoms were primarily identified as reflecting an "Undifferentiated Somatoform Disorder" (DSM-IV-TR 300.82). Even on psychometric assessment, Mary did her best to hide her addiction behind her substantial intelligence and charm. In interviews with me, Mary had likewise been disarming. But, I had been put on the alert both by her history and the fluctuations in her thinking. However, it was not until we received the results of the assessment that I was certain enough about Mary's diagnosis to definitively arrange a confrontation.

Margie: a patient who consistently deceived professionals

In another case, that of Margie, the clinical interviews and assessment were as dramatic as Mary's, but, unlike Mary, testing in that case revealed unexpected psychological health. Margie, from childhood, had been treated as an intellectual and emotional "cripple." She was adopted at birth, the anger and resentment of her adoptive father unchallenged by his compliant wife. Margie's affluent parents covered their disappointment about and hostility toward her by placing her in the finest schools for educationally disabled children. At age 18, she indeed

---

[3] Among the tests used were (1) the Personality Assessment Inventory (PAI) (Morey, 2007), and the Minnesota Multiphasic Personality Inventory (MMPI), both categorized as "personality tests," and (2) the Rorschach test, a "projective," or, more properly, "performance-based" test. All fall within the category of "personality tests," as compared to "neuropsychological tests." In Mary's case all the personality tests used were rife with indications of disabling anxiety and depression.

seemed impaired, acting the role of an immature, intellectually damaged young woman. And yet she was contemptuous and clever in her expression of it; able to get away with her contempt by hiding it behind her apparent intellectual deficiency.

Critical to our purpose, and qualifying this case as "operationally complex," were the multitude of mental health professionals and schools for children with special needs involved in it before and at the time of referral to me (SAF) for a second opinion. Margie, for example, had been tested by educators and psychologists on five occasions. She had been referred twice to well-known, multidisciplinary clinics distant from her home for comprehensive workups. The hope, as expressed by her parents, was that there might be a genetic explanation for her "deficiencies," and that a medical treatment could be found to "correct" her problems.

To make my clinical evaluation, and after contacting physicians and mental heath professionals who had been involved in her care, I met with Margie on six occasions over a period of two months. I found myself intrigued because, although her tendency to talk non-stop could be tedious, I had the sense she was hiding something. The history and clinical interview did not add up, making me wonder whether Margie might be using her disability as a foil to hide hostility toward her adoptive parents. For example, Margie had invented an elaborate story about a boy she claimed was infatuated with her while she was in a boarding school and who was "killed in a skiing accident." The story accumulated extensive detail, and everyone, including Margie's parents and teachers, believed it was real. When I finally asked Margie with confrontational humor whether she might be "bullshitting, and could it be possible that no such event occurred?" she grinned broadly and we both had a belly laugh.

Following the initial sessions we were ready for another assessing psychologist's input. Margie and I formulated our questions. Margie was fervently interested in knowing about the extent of her actual limitations and whether she could ever expect to be considered "normal," have a social life, and hold a job. Clearly, in contrast with Mary whose interest in our work was mostly based on compliance with her parents' wishes, at that point Margie truly wanted help. However, because in a little more than a year Margie was scheduled to leave home for a small college with a program for students with academic limitations, we had a restricted time period in which to do our work.

The psychologist and Margie got on well. Margie appreciated her interest. The psychologist administered the MMPI-2, TAT, Rorschach (Rorschach, 1921), and the Strong (Donnay et al., 2005) and Myers-Briggs Type Indicator Career Report (Myers-Briggs, 1962), as well as the WAIS-III (Wechsler Adult Intelligence Scale) (Wechsler, 1987). Previous assessments had suggested that Margie was cognitively impaired, her verbal and performance IQ apparently barely in the low normal range. However, remarkably, according to the current test battery, her verbal IQ was in the high average range, besting 81% of her peers; her performance score was in the average range, ranking her above 55% of her peers.

Margie was thrilled and even requested a second feedback session with the psychologist. But no one was more surprised, and perhaps dismayed, by the results of the cognitive assessment than Margie's adoptive father, when on every measure of cognition Margie at least equaled her non-impaired peers, her scores all above the mean for a normative cohort of girls of her age and from her background.

In both cases, Mary's and Margie's, feedback meetings to discuss assessment results with the patients and their families enabled me to radically change where our therapeutic interventions needed to be directed.

In the face of the test results, Mary had to admit to her misuse of substances. Mary's addictions, her underlying pessimism, and the defects in her relationship with her much admired mother were exposed in full. Using these findings I worked with Mary for a few months to prepare her for transfer to a drug and alcohol rehabilitation program.

Margie only dared to come out of hiding because she believed I meant her no harm and was genuinely interested in understanding and supporting her. Most likely the startling contrast between the impairment suggested by earlier assessment results and her current assessment emphasizing intellectual competency reflected a combination of Margie's anxiety during test taking and her private reluctance to cooperate with assessments advocated by her adoptive parents. The results of the new test battery were monumental in jump-starting Margie's decision to finally become involved in treatment. Following the current assessment, and after conferring with those who were involved in her treatment, her psychiatric care was transferred to me. After nine months of treatment with me, including the initiation of pharmacotherapy with fluoxetine 20 mg/day to address her anxiety and intermittent depression, Margie went on to a mainstream college. At the time of our last contact she was on track to graduate having maintained a credible academic record.

Postscript

It's hard to imagine medical or psychometric assessment being superfluous to any adequate clinical truing effort. However, as illustrated by Diane, Dorothy, and the numerous cases that need a constant infusion of clinical judgment to stay on target, assessment – psychometric or medical – is also not always the most important guide in the truing process. At times testing of either sort can actually throw a physician off-course, yielding false positives or negatives. The point is that, for any clinical effort to stay on track, multiple truing measures, used in unison and sequentially, are generally required for moving toward an accurate conclusion. With this input, the sources of variance affecting the reliability of the clinical work are progressively reduced. Further, as this complex truing process occurs and unappreciated facets of the patient's problem are uncovered, new truing activities may be revealed and become useful. This assortment of truing measures, as they intersect and correct for each other, serves to cancel out distortions within the clinical process, progressively defining an accurate focus for the treatment.

4

The limitations of algorithms: details of two "clinically complex" treatments

Whether you are a psychiatrist or a PCP, your job is essentially the same. You need to use all the clinical tools at your disposal. You are attempting to account for as much diagnostic and treatment variance as possible, ensuring that the treatments you deliver are the most effective ones. We say "attempting" because, if we could identify all the factors creating your patient's difficulties, we might be able to come up with the best possible interventions every time. But, we can never account for 100% of the problems affecting the patient. There is the opportunistic infection that confounds the most thoughtfully considered antibiotic regimen. There is the crucial "secret" your patient didn't tell you that would have helped in understanding her symptoms.

Truing instruments,[1] the clinical devices through which "truing" is conducted, are one thing. There are plenty of these in medicine; those in systemic medicine presumably no "better," and frequently no different, from those in psychiatry. For example, PCPs and psychiatrists working in medical settings are generally comfortable with direction provided by specialty consultations. This input, the truing it provides, can correct for some of the variance inherent in clinical thinking and add to the "incremental validity" of clinical decisions (also see Chapters 1 and 2 for discussions of the "principle of successive approximations"). "Incremental validity," once again, refers to the increased certainty that accrues as more truing measures are brought into a clinical sequence (Garb, 1984).

---

[1] When referring to "truing" operations the designations "mechanism," "method," "device," "instrument," and "measure" are approximately synonymous. Throughout the text these terms are for the most part used interchangeably. Within limits, however, the selection of which label to employ depends on the context in which it appears, e.g., "mechanism," "measure," "device," or "instrument" is preferred when breaking down diagnostic operations that provide direction for clinical work to their component parts; "method" when referring to a set of procedures. In this text, as often as appropriate, we will stick to the terms "truing method" and "truing measure."

On the other side of the same coin, however, there is the more heavily subjective contribution of "experience-based clinical judgment" (EBCJ), a term we introduced in Chapter 3. Clinical judgment, guided in part by intuition, is always involved as a physician works to arrive at clinical decisions.

Arbitrary factors influencing the choice of truing devices: the example of psychometric assessment

Other, non-technical factors may enter into a clinician's choice of truing instruments, in this instance reducing the reliability of a truing sequence. For example, compare the high frequency with which primary care physicians use medical laboratory tests and diagnostic imaging to the lower probability that a psychiatrist is likely to use psychometric assessment. Since psychometric assessment is among the most powerful truing devices available to psychiatrists, we are impressed that it is not used more routinely. This point has particular validity in the evaluation of complex patients where psychometrics may help in several ways, including: (1) diagnostic specificity, (2) quantification of psychiatric symptoms, and (3) the monitoring of treatment progress.

Full psychometric assessment, however, is generally more costly, less easy to qualify for insurance reimbursement, and more time intensive than a typical panel of blood tests. All of these factors are likely implicated in psychiatrists' frequent choice not to use it. Diagnostic imaging can be expensive too, of course, but, unlike the usual case with psychometric assessment, at least part of its cost is likely to be covered by insurance. Nonetheless, as noted in Chapter 3, it is striking, and perhaps even surprising, that the limited research available about the accuracy of data-supported clinical decisions (Meyer *et al.*, 2001; Meyer, 2003) suggests that psychometric assessment produces information that is about as accurate as laboratory and radiological data.

Decisions

The office: the place where the rubber meets the road. At each clinical moment you, as the physician responsible for treatment, are called on to make decisions, tens of them in each appointment. Since most of these choices are processed automatically, it may be worth stopping for a moment to think back to an actual office visit. Take a half hour interval with your last patient and think about the exact order of events, the choices you had available, and the moves you made. Whoops, so much for a manual laying out the exact steps in treating a particular condition.

Now to clinical practice, the eclectic context in which we as physicians do our work. Evidence-based (EBTs) or empirically supported treatments (ESTs), represented as manualized protocols, reduce clinical problems to syndromes: World Health Organization International Classification of Diseases (ICD-10) or DSM-IV-TR categories that meticulously represent a prototypical patient.

Begin here with psychiatry. Schizoaffective Disorder, as an example, is classified by the ICD-10 into five types: manic, depressive, mixed (manic and depressive), other, and unspecified.

The following are the criteria for diagnosis of a schizoaffective disorder from the *Diagnostic and Statistical Manual of Mental Disorders* (DSM-IV-TR):

(A) Two (or more) of the following symptoms are required to be present for the majority of a one-month period (or a shorter period of time if symptoms got better with treatment):

. delusions;
. hallucinations;
. disorganized speech (e.g., frequent derailment or incoherence) which is a manifestation of formal thought disorder;
. grossly disorganized behavior (e.g., dressing inappropriately, crying frequently) or catatonic behavior;
. negative symptoms: e.g., affective flattening (lack or decline in emotional response), alogia (lack or decline in speech), avolition (lack or decline in motivation), anhedonia (lack or decline in ability to experience pleasure), lack of concentration, or social withdrawal (sometimes called social anhedonia). It should be noted that negative symptoms are different from symptoms of depression.

If the delusions are judged to be bizarre, or hallucinations consist of hearing one voice participating in a running commentary of the patient's actions or of hearing two or more voices conversing with each other, only that symptom is required to meet criterion "A" above. The speech disorganization criterion is only met if it is severe enough to substantially impair communication.

AND at some time during the illness there needs to have been either one, two or all three of the following:

. major depressive episode
. manic episode
. mixed episode.

(B) During the same period of illness, delusions or hallucinations have been present for at least two weeks in the absence of prominent mood symptoms.

(C) Symptoms that meet criteria for a mood episode must have been present for a substantial portion of the total duration of the active and residual periods of the illness.

(D) The disturbance cannot be due to the direct physiological effects of a substance (e.g., a drug of abuse, a medication) or a general medical condition.

Evidence-based treatments (EBTs) for this condition emphasize its chronicity, its tendency to recur over the patient's lifetime, and the centrality of medication in its treatment. The recommended psychotherapy treatment is usually cognitive behavioral therapy (CBT).

The foregoing list of criteria for diagnosing Schizoaffective Disorder is neatly laid out, as are treatment steps incorporated into algorithms for treating this disorder. Frequently, however, these formalized schemas prove inadequate when applied in actual clinical life.

Case illustration: the intersection of diagnosis and temperament

As an example of this kind of divergence, consider John, who was 46 years old and had been diagnosed with schizoaffective disorder. John certainly had periods of distorted thinking associated with episodes of depression. However, he was basically warm and compassionate and could almost always follow a conversation well. He was also a brilliant accountant. It was just that any emotionally charged situation, such as a business partner growing impatient with him, could throw him over the depressive and, at times, mildly thought-disordered edge.

The DSM-IV-TR was certainly helpful in categorizing John's condition and initiating the work with him. But, that was just the start. He was resistant to taking antipsychotic or mood stabilizing medication since those he had previously tried had "dulled" his thinking. He found CBT, for the purpose of revising distorted thought patterns, "simplistic." Medication was nonetheless essential in stabilizing John's mood and disordered thinking. However, what helped him most was the comprehending and directive relationship he developed with his psychiatrist. She seized on and promoted his interest in making friends and caring for his children. Being reminded of these life priorities, reassurance that he had people in his life who loved him and did not just respect his professional achievements, "meant everything" to him.

And what would you as an internist have done about Alan? Following a "standard" treatment protocol for him was soon out of the question. He was diagnosed with myelofibrosis at age 56. His primary medication at first was imatinib. However eventually, and after he developed a potentially fatal medication-induced rash (Stevens–Johnson syndrome), his physicians were forced to rely on interferon. New side effects, including diarrhea, nausea, vomiting, headache, and weight gain, made treatment difficult enough, but Alan refused to change his way of life, substantially complicating his treatment. Late-night carousing continued for as long as he could maintain it. His infidelity alienated his wife, discouraging her from fully cooperating with his medical team. Easing his suffering and prolonging his life through medical management was anything but easy. Confusing to those treating him was that he was likable and always "seemed" to be trying to cooperate.

Discrepancy between standardized expectations of treatment as set down in books and clinical reality is not surprising. As we explicate in Chapter 5, the course of patients' illnesses, as well as the individualized nature of their lives, thinking, emotions, strengths, vulnerabilities, cultural backgrounds, and support systems, establishes a framework of clinical complexity within which treatment occurs.

Illustration of clinical complexity: Alan, a medical and management challenge

A good guy who we all miss. He was a hard-drinking and inveterate gambler. He could be both moody and infinitely generous. Myelofibrosis was diagnosed at age 56. There was no preexisting hematological derangement. He died at the age of 60, leaving three children behind. Born into urban poverty, he created and became wealthy from building his own company selling luxury automobiles.

Alan could be a finagler, a bit sly, not always inclined to tell the truth when it didn't suit him. We couldn't tell, for example, whether Alan had extramarital affairs. He second wife, an exotic Russian woman, insisted that he did, and never let him forget it. Worse, she believed that he was "clearly responsible" for infecting her with genital herpes. From a psychological perspective, it was hard to know how and why a "mover" like Alan would pick a wife like her. Her demonizing of him was unrelenting. And, then there was his deceased wife. She had been taller than him and was inattentive to her appearance. If he was such a "ladies' man," how did he pick this kind of partner for his first mate?

These enigmas introduce this most peculiar and fascinating man. They also provide a background for explaining how poorly he cared for his health, even when he knew how sick he was.

Alan silently, slowly, became sicker, maintaining much of his roguish demeanor until the end. When he was sickest he insisted on getting into his car and driving several thousand miles by himself to visit a relative. Here is where the problem for his physicians came in. While he religiously attended appointments with his university-based hematologist and was reasonably compliant about taking his medication and receiving transfusions, he took risks, mischievously acting against medical advice. He continued his excessive use of alcohol until the last months of his life and regularly exhausted himself with revelry. This was Alan's character, the basis of his successes in business as well as the problems that dogged him in life. He both cooperated and unceasingly cheated; a physician's nightmare since it is so hard in that circumstance to tell why the ostensibly "good" patient is deteriorating. Death came when Alan and his physicians were considering a bone marrow transplant. Sadly that never happened, since over months he became too sick for physicians to risk it. Maybe if he had paid closer attention, but...

Did Alan need psychiatric care to help him stick with his medical treatment regime? Probably a stretch. After all, what would a guy with his inner-city background be doing seeing a "shrink," even after his university-based physicians insisted he see one?

But, nonetheless, he slowly bought in.

The strategy? Simple. Alan understood and craved something he never had been fortunate enough to experience: a good honest commitment from another person, especially someone he respected. In contrast with his experience with the recipients of his never-ending gifts and financial largesse, that person could not want anything material from him. It turned out that few people in Alan's life had ever cared for him without there being strings attached. Generally, what they wanted had something to do with money. In fact, his second wife, the one who reviled him for everything, was explicitly out for just that. She took whatever she could get and still battered him, justifying her malevolence with the claim that he had tricked her into marrying him.

This is where I (SAF) came in. I made every effort to get into Alan's skin, to make myself credible and essential to him. I did this by providing intermittent couples' counseling for Alan and his wife, and, as I became trusted by both of them, accepted their invitation to shift my focus to Alan alone. That suited his wife's purposes since she assumed I could see Alan's alleged iniquity and would deal with it appropriately. Since Alan could actually differentiate between professional and personal motives, and since he quickly found himself liking and trusting me, he jumped on board, incrementally committing himself to the agenda I provided for dealing with his illness and cooperating with his medical team.

Soon the "wife side" of the treatment equation almost disappeared and it was Alan and me working alone. Alan was beginning to open up, discussing his feelings about his disease and asking for more time with me. Ordinarily this development would have provided the leverage to facilitate his obstructed bone marrow transplantation. Sadly, however, it was too late. Over and above the fact that his bone marrow air into together with his red blood cells and platelets, were disappearing, Alan was beginning to develop trouble getting enough, his lungs. The culprit was pulmonary fibrosis, his lungs becoming rigidly bound by scar tissue. He soon required portable oxygen most of the time. His spleen was enlarged and probably needed to be removed. Complications were arising at an alarming rate. Included was the development of leukemia, a frequent end-stage transformation in this condition.

So, Alan decided to do what any "self respecting," terminally ill, inveterate reveler would do. He planned two long, luxurious vacations for himself and his ill-tempered wife. Sadly, she responded in character by gleefully destroying each one of these plans, acting as if they had been contrived to torment her.

Alan died within a few months. He died without fanfare, unable to breathe, the load on his heart increasing until it gave way. By that time he had bequeathed his fortune, fifty million dollars, to his wife who could speak of little more than the herpes he had given her.

Retrospective

What could Alan's medical team, and I as unofficial MPCP, have done?

Our argument is that, by one measure, Alan's, I believe we did pretty well. Alan apparently needed to make up for past sins by taking his wife's abuse and giving her his money. In some twisted way he believed she had come into his life to set him straight. He also needed an unconditional relationship with someone who was dedicated to helping and caring for him. I ultimately provided that. And reform and introspection? Well they were OK. But, not much fun.

By another measure, we failed. Alan's physicians, individually, did their assigned jobs well. His internist made the initial diagnosis and then referred him to university-based hematologists and oncologists, and from there to pulmonologists. Initially, the internist was the *de facto* leader of the team. However, once out of his hands, Alan's medical care was mainly allocated to medical subspecialists. Communication among these physicians was never optimal. Also, while the oncologists and hematologists collaborated with one another, they hardly spoke to Alan and his family. In addition, they never regarded the psychiatrist, myself, as an integral member of the treatment team. Instead, most of his physicians held that the psychiatrist's role was to manage Alan's behavior so he would cooperate with his systemic medical treatment, moving him as quickly as possible to bone marrow transplantation. Alan, on the other hand, would probably have argued that carousing and spending freely until the end was the best way to go.

In sum, then, as we see it, there was one glaring failure in what we believe was a generally adequate treatment. Communication among physicians could have been a lot better. It is likely that, with attention to that source of truing, the course of Alan's illness could have been improved and the pace of his deterioration slowed. With that protection in place, he might even have received the bone marrow transplant he so desperately needed. As unofficial MPCP, I did my best to facilitate communication among his other treating physicians and to have Alan and his wife included in that process, but the effort remained anemic without the full support of his other physicians.

Now, compare Alan to Neal. Neal had systemic medical illnesses, or at least that's what he thought. An internist, an orthopedist, and a neurologist were all part of his clinical team. But, in the end it became clear that his main problems were psychiatric. Our impression, however, is that the parallels between these cases far outweigh the differences. Precision in diagnosis and treatment planning were of overriding importance in both cases. In the illustrations that follow the steps in the development of each case, the truing sequences and the resulting diagnostic and treatment considerations will be emphasized.

Steps in the evolution of a complex case

Neal: a detailed illustration of the truing sequence in a clinically and operationally complex case

How to get lost with a patient in one easy lesson.

Follow carefully: Train for 2, 5, or 10 years – it doesn't really matter how long for this particular exercise. Get an office. Meet the patient for the first time. Get a clear and detailed history, including why the patient is there and the course of his or her difficulties.

Sounds straightforward, doesn't it?[2]

Now, consider Neal, age 22. In the initial phone conversation, Neal was described by his parents as "bright, maybe brilliant, but moody and remarkably stubborn." "He argues with people and gets fired from jobs." "He has plenty of potential but there are lots of reasons why he has left every situation in a puddle of mediocrity." Often these failures followed a breakup with a girlfriend. In high school there was Annabelle, a free spirit who left Neal and moved to Mexico to live with a writer. Dorothy from his first two years of college was more stable but reportedly left Neal because of his "moodiness."

His parents, two well-meaning architects, had singularly focused on Neal's potential for professional success. After all, "his older brother went to Yale, was a model student, and expects to attend medical school."

You begin to build an impression in your mind, looking for diagnostic categories to attach the clinical information you are getting. At this point in the case you may be thinking something like "This is going to be easy. The patient has ADHD. The history supports it." However, after you meet Neal, things become a bit peculiar. He incessantly argues over trivial matters, true. Nonetheless, you are impressed by his personal honesty, as well as his creativity and intelligence.

So, now you are beginning to get lost. Of course, you can attempt to avoid confusion by depending on your current diagnostic impression and prescribing medication, something like methylphenidate for ADHD or lamotrigine for his mood disorder. But, what precisely are you targeting? And how far-reaching and lasting are the results likely to be?

Regarding psychotherapy, you mention CBT to him since that seems like an obvious next step. He's OK with the idea, but, to your dismay, he says he's tried CBT and found it "uninteresting and unhelpful."

What to do at this point? What outline, what algorithms, to follow? What exactly are you treating?

Step by step recounting of the truing sequence as it unfolded with Neal

Here is a condensed, albeit nonetheless detailed recounting of the steps I (SAF) followed as I evaluated Neal. It is presented in a way that highlights the multitude of factors that had to be considered at each point, as well as their shifting nature.

Impression of the patient (the first truing step in this clinical evaluation)

Awkward and disheveled, Neal looked like he belonged in a Paris garret, spending his time drinking absinthe with other intellectuals and talking about philosophy.

---

[2] Collecting background information is, of course, an essential part of every initial workup. Our procedure, in addition to requesting reports from other involved professionals, the patient, and parents, if the patient is a child, includes the patient or parent filling out an extensive background questionnaire. Gathering data in this manner saves time and increases efficiency.

History of the present illness (taking an initial history, truing step 2)

Neal was referred to me (SAF) after he was dismissed from college for the second time in three years. Since he was a superior student in high school and such a good thinker, he was admitted to an excellent private college. He was expelled, however, after getting drunk and protesting an administrative decision affecting his girlfriend by driving his beat-up automobile recklessly around the campus police station while screaming epithets. This episode was one of many where Neal became implicated in outrageous behavior. He then transferred to a state college but had to take a leave of absence after a year because he failed to do his academic work. By the point of referral, his parents were feeling so defeated in their attempt to deal with his failures that they were willing to let me "do anything to retrieve the essential Neal."

Initial contact and review of records (truing step 3)

Here is what I did from the point of referral. I had a long telephone call with Neal's parents and told them that I would see Neal for an evaluation. With his permission I would then meet with them as well. I would want to see copies of his school records and whatever psychometric assessment reports they could get. In conjunction with taking a history, I would ask them and Neal to fill out an extensive background information form.

Excerpts from the initial interview with Neal and the clinical evaluation (truing steps 4 and 5)

Neal's mental status examination was largely unremarkable. He was as moody and reluctant to cooperate as his parents reported. "Nothing is wrong," he claimed, outside of his "parents' heavy handedness and their excessive worry." But, he had "no choice," so he said he would continue to meet with me.

At first he minimized virtually all his problems including his school failures. He did tell me, however, that he had been having headaches, as well as neck and back pain, and had experienced intermittent blurred vision and "flashes of light," making him concerned he might have a neurological disorder.

Psychometric (psychological and/or neuropsychological) assessment (truing step 6)

A neurological workup and of psychometric assessment was in order. However, why go to all the trouble and expense to get a formal psychometric assessment? The initial cost was to be, at minimum, $3000. But, think about the information that would be missing with a "bare bones" approach, using only clinical observation. Think of the wasted time and expense if Neal were to find himself in "off target" treatment.

The initial intervention, medication, and treatment plan ("truing step")

Based on the history and my initial impression, it would have been easy enough to conclude that Neal suffered mainly from ADHD. In that case, prescribing a psychostimulant might have been appropriate.

But that was far from the whole picture (truing step 4 above, obtaining additional clinical history) From the point of view of temperament, Neal's stubbornness and objections to being scrutinized were uncompromising. In terms of developmental influences, there was his father's heart attack when Neal was nine and his older brother's high level of performance – a standard to which Neal was always compared. Add, repeated school failures and several peculiar "dyscontrol" episodes like the one that got him expelled from college, as well as the history of headaches, neck and back pain, and visual symptoms. Also, Neal used alcohol rather freely and perhaps abusively. On the positive side were Neal's intelligence and capacity for creativity, although even these attributes were a bit obscured by how easily he became frustrated when people and situations did not meet his standards and expectations. To begin with I prescribed amphetamine plus dextroamphetamine (in the form of Adderall). Neal participated in the treatment planning (truing step seven, setting the initial treatment contract, as well as attempting to identify tentative outcome measures) and, in accordance with his wishes, we set the frequency of sessions to an hour and a half every other week. As mentioned, the prospect of psychometric assessment, in this case both personality and neuropsychological assessment, was introduced early in treatment, but it required eight months of treatment before Neal agreed to it together with an associated neurological workup.

Neuropsychological assessment and neurological workup (truing step 8, additional medical and psychometric assessments)

As you know, Neal worried about his health. He had a suspicion that his abuse of alcohol might have caused some brain damage. With this concern in mind, he ultimately embraced the idea that a neurological workup and associated medical tests might provide information addressing these concerns.

The neurological examination, together with a brain Magnetic resonance image (MRI) and x-rays of Neal's spine, proved to be entirely normal. Even his cervical spine was within normal limits – a finding leaving the source of his frequent headaches obscure. The neuropsychological assessment, however, underscored the seriousness of Neal's ADHD, and, together with the personality testing, identified a temperamental idiosyncrasy characterized by emotional reactivity and a marked tendency to brood. While irritability is frequently associated with ADHD, there was still something we did not understand about Neal's behavioral peculiarities. As a result, we decided to undertake additional, more extensive, personality testing.

Further psychometric assessment (optional truing step 9, additional personality testing and a second opinion from a new psychologist)

Thus far our treatment team consisted of a neurologist, a neuropsychologist, and an orthopedist, in addition to myself, a psychiatrist. At this point, for the extended personality testing, we were joined by Philip Erdberg (PE), another psychologist who had special expertise in "performance based" assessment (traditionally referred to as "projective testing"). Soon thereafter, one additional psychologist who specialized in CBT for the treatment of ADHD also joined the team.

In contrast to the first testing psychologist's findings, PE's take on the situation emphasized Neal's unique assets, most particularly his unusual and distinctly unconventional intellect and creativity. As was stated in the narrative section of Dr. Erdberg's report, "Neal gets bored easily, excluding him from the class of people who, like his brother, can sit still for four years of college. Neal insists on being starkly independent and becomes infuriated when anyone encroaches on his privacy. This impatience, however, unlike that typical of ADHD, appears to be substantially predicated on Neal's brilliance and his intolerance of commonplace experience."

In consonance with this view, it had also become apparent in treatment sessions that, to guard his autonomy, Neal lived in a way that was remarkably unrealistic. Cheese sandwiches were fine for breakfast, lunch, and dinner, just so long as no one was forcing an agenda down his throat and he could do what truly interested him. Somehow he would get money for his other needs. He could get bored at a moment's notice. This propensity set up a vicious cycle. Neal would stay with a situation for a short while, get impatient, and immediately have to move on, if for no other reason than to create stimulation for himself.

And, there was no reason why Neal's response to the psychometric assessments and psychiatric treatment would be any exception. Even if I could manage to get Neal engaged in treatment there was every reason to expect that he would soon become impatient with that process and quit.

What would you have done in this situation (truing step 10, decision about how to proceed: formulation of a treatment plan arrived at collaboratively with the patient)?

Would you have maintained a regular liaison with Neal's parents with the partial purpose of facilitating Neal's adherence to treatment, as I did? When recommending or providing psychotherapy would you, as his psychotherapist during high school, have selected an insight-oriented approach or recommended CBT instead?

What would the outcome have been if it had just been Neal and me working together, leaving out the parents? One likely answer is that his parents would have remained overly compliant with Neal's demands and not insisted that Neal cooperate for long enough for a meaningful course of treatment to take shape. His usual pattern would likely have repeated, with Neal getting interested for at best a short period and then becoming bored and quitting.

How to do it (truing step 10 continued: the treatment plan)

Don't get bound to protocol. Do that and you may well lose the patient's interest and commitment and, thus, fail.

In Alan's situation this requirement was incontestable. He engineered multiple deflections from appropriate treatment, determining that requirements for compliance with treatment be regularly readjusted to accommodate his idiosyncratic preferences.

Neal, except for his ADHD diagnosis, did not fit into any conventional diagnostic category. Algorithms were unable to encompass the clinical complexity I encountered as I began to work with him. Apart from using my clinical judgment, how then did I determine Neal's diagnosis and identify a viable approach to his treatment?

Physician self-monitoring

At this point, we want to bring in physician self-monitoring – devices for tracking progress in treatment (truing step eleven: physician self-monitoring).

In systemic medicine this part of the work generally consists of repeat laboratory tests, diagnostic imaging, and consultations with other physicians. Similar determinations are available in psychiatry, but less likely to be used as broadly.

There are, of course, other methods for following clinical progress, including those that depend on clinical observation (Garb, 1984; Atlas, 2009). In Chapter 5 we will describe a practical self-monitoring method we call the *Self-Other Rapid Assessment Method* ("SO Method") and its application the *Self-Other Rapid Assessment Analysis* ("SO Analysis"). The framework on which this assessment device is based breaks down the physician's clinical observations into a handful of personality-associated categories that, along with other applications, can be used to assess the patient's ability to adhere to treatment.

The "descriptive distillation" given below of Neal's clinical status toward the end of his evaluation is in part derived from a series of "SO analyses" done to assess his ability to be productively involved in treatment. A more detailed "SO analysis" of Neal, done at a later point during his treatment, will be given in the next chapter following an explanation of this assessment method and how it works.

Descriptive distillation: what do we have so far?
Who actually *was* Neal?

Exquisitely vulnerable to social ostracism, intolerant and irritable, gifted and morally upright, Neal lacked social refinement and adequate social judgment. He was also rigid, unable to entertain much feedback that he considered judgmental, and impatient when things didn't go his way. At age 22 he was about as resilient as a sea anemone that pulls in its tentacles whenever touched. Worse, he didn't easily acknowledge these vulnerabilities and was loath to discuss them in any depth. So, while ADHD may have been a prominent factor in determining his behavior, in Neal's case his psychology and adjustment problems gain special prominence.

The problem side of Neal, as you already know, was paired with his intellectual gifts. Neal could see deeper and farther into cognitively complex problems than almost any other 22-year-old with whom I (SAF) have worked. When he could swallow his pride for long enough and apply for jobs, he almost always was hired. To the extent he was willing to stay with a job he did surprisingly well. When he signed up for graphic design classes at the local community college, he captured the imagination of all of his teachers.

So we're back to a "fish out of water," Adjustment Disorder (DSM-IV-TR 309.9, Adjustment Disorder, Unspecified) formulation of Neal's psychopathology. Neal could easily and accurately see other people's deficits. He tended to be incisive in these judgments. What he couldn't acknowledge were his own shortcomings.

Step by step recounting of the truing sequence with Neal, continued Neal's diagnosis (truing step 12, the tentative assignment of a diagnosis)

In addition to meeting the criteria for an Adjustment Disorder (DSM-IV-TR 309.9, Adjustment Disorder, Unspecified), diagnostically Neal conformed to all of the following formal and descriptive categories.

(1) Depression: certainly Neal was prone to bouts of depression, lasting from days to weeks. His temperamental status, however, was best characterized as consisting of a chronic gray mood and irritability, perhaps qualifying him for the diagnosis "Dysthymic Disorder DSM-IV-TR 300.4." But precisely what kinds of mood disturbances were these, and how much of his chronic moroseness was due to temperament, indelible consequences of his neurobiology? To what extent are "awkward," "shy," or "moody," all adjectives describing Neal's behavior, discrete psychological maladies?

(2) Attention-Deficit/Hyperactivity Disorder (ADHD), DSM-IV-TR 314.01: we have already considered this category, and clearly ADHD seems like a correct diagnostic designation for Neal. However, we need to throw you off center a bit again. Neal's response to the 12 cognitive behavioral sessions for dealing with ADHD led the psychologist who administered these to suggest that his was an "unusual" sort of ADHD since it yielded so readily to the behavioral protocol she used and did not seem to limit Neal's capacity for creativity.

(3) How about a Personality Disorder (Axis II, DSM-IV-TR), namely (a) a variation of a Paranoid Personality Disorder, distinguished by "Passive-Aggressive Features" (301.0 DSM-IV-TR), or (b) even a variant of a Schizoid

Personality Disorder (301.20 DSM-IV-TR)? To be considered in this category, in addition to biology is the effect of early and ongoing experience. While it was natural for Neal's parents to appreciate his brother who apparently breezed through social and academic challenges, they may have been consistently offended by Neal's temperamentally based standoffishness. The mismatch between Neal and themselves could have begun early in Neil's life, creating chronic misattunement between himself and his parents. In fact both explanations seem cogent, suggesting that biology and experience could have worked in concert and have been implicated in creating Neal's self-esteem and social, as well as behavioral, problems.

(4) Intelligence and creativity: as you know, Neal was a brilliant thinker. He insisted on being "unconventional," however, and needed to be constantly stimulated. It certainly would have been easy for people to misunderstand Neal as he was growing up, confusing his unusual cognitive requirements for his being "limited," "odd," or "troubled."

Physician decisions and actions (truing step 13: decisions about how to proceed)

As Neal's treating physician what would you have done? Let's break it down.

(1) In-depth, focused, psychodynamic psychotherapy to help Neal understand the nature of his difficulties and work them through was obviously in order. Neal had never been willing to sit still long enough to reflect on why, with all his assets, he repeatedly failed in life. The key here is that Neal's personal accessibility was so limited. Probing for the sake of clarifying the nature of Neal's problems and advice had to be dosed carefully so Neal could take in what was said. These interventions had to be strategized so Neal would experience them as friendly and, ideally, internalize the associated insights as if they were his own. Nothing, but nothing, that other people said could be accepted *a priori*.

(2) Psychoeducation about how to understand and handle ADHD: this instruction was made available as 12 weekly sessions and proved quite useful. One objective for this training was to acquaint Neal with the manifestations of his ADHD and its likely course. Neal's impatience and moodiness were never absent as he undertook this project and, in fact, became a subject for the training itself.

(3) Medication: Neal was reliably self-observant about the effects of medication. He reported that adding a psychostimulant helped him to control his moods and concentrate. He experienced little benefit, however, from sertraline, a selective serotonin re-uptake inhibitor (SSRI), prescribed to address his anxiety and depression.

(4) Additional psychotherapy, in this case a separate course of CBT to provide guidance for Neal about social propriety, as well as about the nature and interpersonal impact of his defensiveness. These issues needed to be dealt

with *in vivo*, as they came up. At each point of experienced or anticipated failure Neal became irritable and withdrew into distracting personal projects, or turned to video games and alcohol for relief.

(5) Ongoing guidance for Neal's parents: Neal's parents wanted to help him, but their behavior, while well-intentioned, was often ill-conceived. They continued to compare Neal to his brother, focus too heavily on their desire that Neal finish college, and were altogether too enmeshed in his correcting his "deviant" lifestyle. Orchestrating this part of the intervention was tricky. Neal, of course, needed to know that I was talking with his parents. However, there was a risk that my involvement with them would reinforce Neal's tendency to blame them for his problems. Also, my speaking with his parents could easily be seen by Neal as a violation of his confidentiality. My solution was always to limit parent telephone calls and meetings to a minimum, decreasing them as Neal became progressively committed to our work.

One idiosyncratic and risky part of this clinical strategy was my support for his parents' requirement that, to continue to receive their financial support, Neal had to remain in psychiatric treatment until its reasonable conclusion. At first Neal's resistance about complying with this condition was powerful. He kept insisting that he wanted, indeed "needed" to join his friends in a distant state. But, with my encouragement the parents held firm, mandating that Neal had to "sit still" for at least the rest of the academic year and bring therapy to a reasonable conclusion, or there would be no funding.

(6) Team coordination: the multiple physicians and psychologists involved in Neal's treatment needed to be consulted and organized as his treatment evolved. This, of course, was my job as MPCP.

(7) Clinical judgment: no one part of this intervention could have been entirely preplanned or prioritized. In Neal's case, each component was brought in as Neal became ready for it. The results of the neuropsychological and personality assessments helped us to orchestrate this process, but clinical judgment, intuition, and clinical experience had to be our primary guides. When I lost sight of what Neal was feeling and what he needed in the moment, we could easily lose direction.

Summary

Amphetamine plus dextroamphetamine 20 mg twice daily worked well for Neal, while sertraline even at 40 mg/day had no visible effect on his depressed mood or anxiety. In-depth, focused, individual psychodynamic and directive psychotherapy was also clearly helpful. Cognitive behavioral therapy (CBT) favorably impacted his ADHD, and collateral work with Neal's parents, as well as personal guidance for Neal, provided the structure and direction he required to progress.

Generalizations

As in most real-life clinical situations, diagnosis and treatment with both Alan and Neal emerged as remarkably complex clinical undertakings. It would have been convenient had there been algorithms, evidence-based treatment protocols, to entirely guide us through each treatment. But, even then, how could they incorporate Alan's personal requirement for both a committed relationship with and admiration from his physicians, as well as his need for mischief and levity as a condition for compliance with medical treatment? And, where to place Neal's social anxiety in the decision tree, since it was not central to his clinical picture? How would an EBT anticipate Alan's repeated defections from proper treatment or Neal's mixed irritability and brilliance? Recall that much of Neal's ADHD-like impatience, when scrutinized, could actually be framed as "frustrated brilliance?"

Add to the above the question of how much of one's behavior is explained by training and culture. In Alan's case there was his culturally and financially impoverished early life; in Neal's, his parents' uncomplimentary comparison of him with his older brother as at least one contribution. These environmental and developmental factors usually play a limited role in evidence-based treatment protocols. There are also intangible personality characteristics, categories of resilience and vulnerability, explaining why some people prevail in difficult circumstances and others do not. Also, when we focus on a patient's problems are we inclined to underestimate assets? Finally, there are physician-originated artifacts, introduced into treatment as departures from standard treatment protocols and potentially altering the clinical process. Examples in these two cases include the possible effects on evaluation and treatment of SAF's unconventional decision to work regularly with Alan's wife early in that treatment, and, in Neal's case, his choice to collaborate with Neal's parents.

The MPCP

Neither Alan's nor Neal's treatment was a one-physician operation. In both cases, a treatment team, organized and supervised by a psychiatrist (SAF) functioning as an MPCP, provided the breadth to make the comprehensive treatment effective. With Alan, however, the inability of his university-based physicians to find the time and motivation to collaborate with SAF on a regular basis established limitations for that treatment. Nonetheless, SAF's liaison with Alan's wife and intermittent consultations with each of his university-based physicians enabled a limited team-like effort to occur.

The complexity continues, however. In Neal's case, SAF's collaborative work with his parents was required for them to support and yet not interfere with his treatment. SAF's alliance with the psychologists and neurologist who were ultimately engaged in that treatment allowed for a conjoint approach to formulating

Neal's diagnoses and for confronting Neal with the reality of their existence. In both treatments, Alan's and Neal's, SAF's credibility with professional members of the treatment team was fundamental for making the treatments work.

The next chapter

In the next chapter, dealing with how the complex nature of the clinical field affects treatment decisions, we will discuss the *SO Rapid Assessment Method* and its contribution to making an immediate appraisal of a clinical situation. From moment to moment the ground rules of any treatment shift; at points leaving physician and patient in a momentary therapeutic daze, disconcerted by clinical complexity and subjectivity. That subjectivity comes from three sources: the physician, the patient, and the two attempting to understand one another. Please don't imagine that the physician and patient by themselves can always reliably sort out the uncertainties of their interpersonal situation. At times they can do pretty well in spite of the restrictions in their ability to make fully objective judgments. But soon they may reach their limits, disagreement and disjunction (Frankel, S., 2000) becoming apparent. Yet, if they can be sufficiently reflective, that is the point at which they may be prompted to modify their assumptions about the treatment, revise their treatment plan, and, when appropriate, enlist a consultant.

5

Negotiating the subjectivity and inter-subjectivity of the clinical field: the complexity inherent in clinical work

Start with a random, rather typical psychiatric office visit. The presenting problems seem straightforward enough. I (SAF) have just taken a history from a new patient, a 43-year-old man. He tells me he's been so depressed that he "can hardly work" and is "arguing with almost everyone."

I continue: "However, our work may touch on some additional, problematic areas you may not have anticipated. As you expect, your Armenian background and strong family ties are likely to be issues. You believe you still have a hard time getting beyond your parents' expectation that you should have married an Armenian woman. You say you also worry incessantly about your 12-year-old daughter who has Limb-Girdle Muscular Dystrophy (LGMD). She is refusing to go to school on some days because other children are beginning to tease her. Her need for medical care and the attention she requires also seem to be impacting your eight-year-old son who is now having temper tantrums. Oh, and what's that about your business being slow?"

Suddenly the playing field is getting complicated. Given all the factors that need to be considered, how do we pick and choose which to take on and in what order? What is the central, inciting issue, or, as in most cases, issues? Which of these does the patient need to understand in depth, and which problems can he cope with independently? Does psychotropic medication make sense, especially since he says he has tried them on several occasions and the side effects have been more troublesome than the therapeutic benefits?

Solomon

It is no different in systemic medicine than in psychiatry: straightforward diagnostic impressions expanding into multiple diagnoses, medication side effects intervening, unexpected personal and interpersonal complications impeding treatment.

Solomon's situation is of interest here. He was 65 and had received the diagnosis of scleroderma at age 50. He was frightened, but could understand the disease well enough given his background as a physical therapist. At age 55 there was a hip replacement and then, at age 60, another hip replacement that did not work very well. Complicating it all was that his wife had filed for divorce four months earlier, abruptly leaving him for a second cousin.

When I (SAF) met Solomon, the wear and tear caused by his medical and personal situation was striking. Once quite handsome, the originally slow-moving cutaneous lesions, now infected and progressively affecting his arms, fingers, feet, and finally his face, made him look hideous. As a result of the scleroderma and arthritic hip degeneration, his ambulation was severely restricted, making it necessary for him to use an electric vehicle to get around. His esophagus had been affected, creating difficulty swallowing, severe gastrointestinal reflux, and making TPN (total parenteral nutrition) feedings necessary. He also had started to develop some difficulty breathing; an ominous sign of lung involvement. Add to this picture the grinding depression that had afflicted Solomon since his wife's departure.[1]

Nonetheless, Solomon managed. True, he limited his social contacts and now spent much of his time watching TV. But, his mind was sharp and his attitude matter-of-fact. He was complex and simple at the same time. The way Solomon put it was, "This is the way things are and I'll do my life now in the best way I know how to. No need for whining." Or at least that's how it was until his son and daughter-in-law became involved. They contacted me saying that Solomon needed help, adding that he was "indulging himself" and required a "good shove from a psychiatrist to get back on his feet."

Clinical complexity mandates strategy

Like it or not, given the complicated nature of most clinical situations and the need to plan and prioritize our interventions, we find ourselves seizing on the word "strategy." For some of us "strategy" may be synonymous with "manipulation," a word suggesting that the physician is somehow tricking the patient into making particular choices. Our position is quite the opposite. We hold that all practitioners constantly make strategic choices whether or not these are acknowledged.

Many physicians don't bother much with deliberate strategizing. Explaining and educating are integrated into their treatments, but once informed about the physician's impression and plan, patients are expected to comply. If not, it's his

---

[1] Solomon's scleroderma was initially diagnosed 15 years earlier as "limited cutaneous scleroderma." Over time, systemic involvement became obvious, the disease affecting Solomon's gastrointestinal tract and eventually his lungs. Since there are no treatments for scleroderma itself, each area of involvement had to be managed separately (Gabrielli *et al.*, 2009).

or her folly. The physician doesn't have time for many tentative moves in creating and implementing a treatment strategy, and these detours may be viewed by the physician as problematic, impeding the pace of treatment.

In systemic medicine, strategy refers to the timing and prioritizing of treatment interventions. The physician chooses which interventions should be emphasized and when, as well as what measures to use to accurately assess the patient and move the treatment along as efficiently as possible. However, in psychiatry, "strategy" may have the unfortunate connotation of pulling the wool over the patient's eyes, unbalancing the interpersonal field in favor of the psychiatrist's control and authority (Greenberg, 1986, 1999; Hoffman, 1996; Mitchell, 1997).

But, what about negotiating a treatment alliance (Norcross, 2002; Hilsenroth & Cromer, 2007; Zeber *et al.*, 2011), an item almost always fundamental to a successful treatment strategy? Look at any list of "core competencies" taught in medical education. Respect for the patient, leading to a sound working relationship, is never missing. Witness the following list of core competencies from the University of Texas Health Science Center at San Antonio (updated April 18, 2008), and pay special attention to the items where we've placed asterisks: www. anesthesia.uthscsa.edu/Residency/ACGMECoreCompetencies.

The ACGME (Accreditation Council for Graduate Medical Education) dictates that residency programs require residents to develop competencies in the six areas below to the level expected of a new practitioner. Toward this end, programs must define the specific knowledge, skills, and attitudes required and provide educational experiences as needed in order for their residents to demonstrate:

Patient Care that is compassionate, appropriate, and effective for the treatment of health problems and the promotion of health.

Medical Knowledge about established and evolving biomedical, clinical, and cognate (e.g., epidemiological and social-behavioral) sciences and the application of this knowledge to patient care.

Practice-Based Learning and Improvement that involves investigation and evaluation of their own patient care, appraisal and assimilation of scientific evidence, and improvements in patient care.

Interpersonal and Communication Skills that result in effective information exchange and teaming with patients, their families, and other health professionals.

Professionalism, as manifested through a commitment to carrying out professional responsibilities, adherence to ethical principles, and sensitivity to a diverse patient population.

Systems-Based Practice, as manifested by actions that demonstrate an awareness of and responsiveness to the larger context and system of health care and the ability to effectively call on system resources to provide care that is of optimal value.

The asterisked items are never missing from a contemporary list of fundamental skills expected of physicians. This is an admirable development in medical education, acknowledging the contribution of the patient, his or her cooperation and attitude, to the success of the treatment. But, how often do physicians consciously emphasize these skills as they move along in their careers? Our impression is that, as clinical requirements become more pressing, the more subtle psychological and interpersonal elements tend to be regarded as more discretionary than most of the other competencies. Physicians are always well-meaning. But, they are often too busy and too much under the press of clinical, financial, and legal considerations to stick to the "old country physician" model, where psychosocial aspects of care were routinely prioritized (Berwick, 2008).

The ideal: the division of responsibility in treatment

To what extent can and should responsibility in treatment be balanced, with the clinician and patient each contributing their part? This most intriguing question is asked routinely by those interested in the nature and quality of the clinician–patient, in our case physician–patient, relationship (Roter, 2000; Norcross, 2002; Frankel, R., 2004; Gelso, 2009) and on a more theoretical level by "inter-subjectively" oriented psychologists. These theoreticians maintain a clinical focus bounded by the bi-personal nature of the clinical relationship and the subjectivity of both participants, patient and clinician (Aron, 1996; Mitchell, 1997, 1998; Hoffman, 1998; Mitchell & Aron, 1999; Stolorow *et al.*, 2002; also see Frankel, S., 2008). According to them, all experience, whether in a personal or clinical setting, is constituted of interacting personal "fields," with the product reflecting the interplay of at least two differently organized experiential worlds.

Framed in this way, the reaching for areas of shared understanding and consensus is an essential objective of all clinical work. It may be worth noting, however, that the consensus referred to is achieved through the intentional process of interpersonal collaboration, while "inter-subjectivity," bilateral interpersonal influence, is a state of being that automatically characterizes all human interactions (Orange *et al.*, 1997). Nonetheless, when all is said and done, even inter-subjectively oriented theoreticians conclude that full parity, the equivalence of influence between physician and patient, is ultimately an unrealistic objective for clinical work (Hoffman, 1998; Mitchell & Aron, 1999). In the final analysis, the clinician, a physician in our case, is ultimately responsible for creating and enforcing structure in this co-created treatment situation.

Unfortunately, except for its place in their medical school and residency curriculum, our impression is that the subject of collaboration between physician and patient is likely to be given limited attention by practicing physicians. We are sure many of these physicians would be happy to accord the patient a more central place in clinical matters. Few, however, are likely to remain interested in it as a riveting topic or find much time to think much about it as they pursue their busy practices.

Contaminating factors

Further interfering with the development of a satisfactory bond between physician and patient, and generally hidden behind both the physician's and patient's ostensibly good intentions, are private ambitions and biases creating unstated agendas within treatment. If the patient were the only one introducing these contaminants the situation might be simple. However, they are as likely to be brought in by the physician. For the record, the traditional labels for two of the most familiar of these "agendas" are "transferences" and "countertransferences." When these come into play in the clinical interaction they are called "enactments."

Why use the word "agendas" and not stick to traditional terminology? Are we simply replacing one set of definitions with another? The answer is convoluted, based in the complexity of any interpersonal exchange. "Transference" refers to the insertion into a current relationship of interactional prototypes carried over from the patient's earlier life. "Countertransference" refers to the same kind of mental activity, but instead introduced by the physician. However, it isn't that simple. Clinical interactions are made up of so many parts, some subtle and others straightforward, that a cartographer would be baffled about how to "map" them. Hence, transferences and countertransferences are likely to only be a fraction of the physician's and the patient's extra-therapeutic contributions to their interaction.

How, then, does this breakdown apply to systemic medicine? Think about it. Can you really imagine a primary care physician or specialist who is entirely free of personal agendas and opinions about proper treatment? Alan's main hematologist was fervent about finding ways to contain and manage Alan's myelodysplasia.[2] His internist, who had known Alan longer than had the hematologist, however, was a bit fed up with Alan. She had less tolerance than the hematologist did for "uncooperative" patients. She had also come to distrust Alan, seeing him as a bit "sleazy," as did his wife. The hematologist and the internist also had somewhat different medical philosophies about how to manage myelodysplasia: which medications to use and when, at which point to remove the spleen, the odds of a bone marrow transplant succeeding, and how to balance the risks of transplant failure against Alan's anticipated longevity without a transplant. So far we have the influence of two physicians' personality traits, their idiosyncratic reactions to the patient, and their differing medical philosophies about Alan's treatment.

---

[2] Myelodysplastic syndromes are clonal abnormalities of marrow cells characterized by varying degrees of cytopenias effecting one or more cell lines. The prognosis is defined by the marrow blast percentage, karyotype and cell lineage affected. Allogeneic bone marrow transplantation is the only curative therapy, with a 60% success rate for those young enough to tolerate the procedure (*Harrison's Principles of Internal Medicine*, 17th edition, Fauci *et al.*, 2008).

Who leads?

Of the named factors shaping the clinical situation, there is one that especially merits emphasis. Someone has to lead. The patient has come to seek advice and direction from a trained and experienced professional, in this case a physician. No matter how you cut it, that person is responsible for treatment outcome. The patient's welfare is in his or her hands. So, however much you are committed to the principle of reciprocity in the clinical work, the physician's role is always magnified by his or her expertise and authority. This power and its attendant responsibility has its potential pitfalls, however. As an example, it can be license for the physician to express his or her biases in the form of excessive control and authority (Haug & Lavin, 1979; Renik, 1993; May, 1995; Mitchell, 1998; Greenberg, 1999; Winblad, 2008). To minimize this possibility, physicians need to be assiduous in monitoring their behavior and remaining open to feedback from their patients.

Strategy versus responsibility for results

Return to the value of reciprocity: shared influence and responsibility between physician and patient. If you hold to that principle, isn't the notion of assuming unchallenged leadership and being strategic in treatment a corruption? Yes and no. Obviously, if you as the physician in charge believe in the ideal of clinical reciprocity, you need to be meticulous about maintaining an authentic, and thoroughly respectful, collaborative atmosphere in treatment. But, as emphasized above, you also have the responsibility of making sure the treatment stays on course.

How then to reconcile these two apparently contradictory points of view? Our opinion is that the physician's ability to maintain these two attitudes simultaneously is actually a requirement, not an option, for successful treatment. Being clinically strategic does not necessarily mandate that the physician neglect any vital interpersonal consideration. To be fully effective, strategy in clinical work needs to be rooted in both the physician's authenticity and competence. The bottom line in treatment, however, will always be whether the patient trusts and respects the physician (Frankel, R., 2004; Frankel, R. & Inui, 2006). After all, what human being would "really" listen to another if these qualities were absent?

Back now to the question of how physicians can simultaneously guard this authenticity and remain strategic nonetheless. To find at least part of the answer, consider the longitudinal course of treatment. The patient, after months of a productive treatment, may not be the same person he or she was at the start, and as treatment moves along it may not remain as necessary for the physician to remain as deliberately strategic in orchestrating clinical interventions.

Neal's treatment offers a good example of this principle. Treatment with me (SAF) couldn't have gotten off the ground without his parents insisting that he "bite the bullet," remain in treatment, and do something personally constructive with his life. They were adamant and tied their financial support to this requirement. Neal had never been in psychiatric treatment before and had no idea whether it could help him. It turns out that they were right to insist on their conditions. Had they not, he almost certainly would have left treatment prematurely. After months of work, however, believe it or not, Neal and I were working like two peas in a pod, managing beautifully together. He came to trust me, increasingly wanting to progress in life and school, in effect confirming the value of the strategy we had used.

Alan, of course, did not really cooperate with any of his physicians until I came along and gave him a prominent part in orchestrating his treatment. Unfortunately, his other physicians, while supportive of our work, failed to grasp the profound importance of involving Alan in a similar way.

How do these "patient-centered" principles, therapeutic reciprocity, with a significant part of the responsibility for keeping the treatment moving along accruing to the patient, bear on the role of the MPCP? From the start, the MPCP is accountable for elaborating the mission of the treatment. In addition to whatever direct clinical services he or she provides, the MPCP makes sure the patient's initiative is preserved and encouraged throughout the treatment, and that the involved physicians utilize the patient as a clinical ally. The place of the patient as a collaborating member of the treatment team needs to be continually reaffirmed. Absent this reinforcement, the patient's voice may be lost as treatment moves along.

Clinical intuition versus strategy

Return to the complexity of the physician's clinical role. Strategy, especially if the physician is experienced, frequently isn't given a great deal of *intentional* consideration as physician and patient move from point to point in their work. At least in part, that aspect of the clinical process feels and looks intuitive. However, as you will see later in this chapter, decisions based on clinical intuition are often more deliberate, more strategic, than they appear from the surface.

So, we're waffling. We are taking the position that clinical work is complex and technically demanding, and that nonetheless it is equally legitimate for a physician to lean on intuition.

We may have just disqualified ourselves with the "hard thinkers" among us. Actually, like them, we believe it behooves all physicians to hold to that which is empirically supported, is as much as possible devoid of assertion and subjectivity. At the same time, the place of experience and judgment in informing the clinical process cannot be minimized.

Our bottom line position is that few interpersonally constituted efforts with the objective of symptom resolution or modification of personality disorders are fully reducible to evidence-based formulas (Novotny & Thompson-Brenner, 2004; Westen & Bradley, 2005; Fonagy, 2006). The ground rules frequently shift as the needs, mood, and opinions of the two people engaged in the treatment evolve. Alterations of various sorts, positive and negative, are unavoidable in ongoing clinical work.

What, then, is the proper mix of these two extremes, the intuitive-interpersonal versus the deliberately strategic, for making a treatment work? Let's look back at Neal. How did I (SAF) know early in treatment to bring Neal's parents into the work? And, what encouraged me to remain positive about someone as rejecting and, at times, morose as Neal? How about the timing of my finally introducing disciplined introspection into our work, for example, by encouraging Neal to look at the effect of having to compete with an always successful older brother who was distinctly more ambitious than he? These and numerous other considerations governed my behavior with Neal. As with any clinical formula that works, the mixture of factors, the balance of clinical judgment and deliberate strategy, often changed from meeting to meeting.

Could I have used a standard protocol for treatment of Dysthymic Disorder, Major Depression, ADHD, or Social Anxiety Disorder with Neal? Yes and no. In fact, I used all four, but only as long they made sense to Neal and me. As well, amphetamine plus dextroamphetamine helped with behavioral regulation. From that point, encouraging him to be more socially active made a difference. Cognitive behavioral therapy for ADHD gave him tools for being more patient and purposeful. Neal found the neuropsychological and personality assessments to be interesting and useful, and was relieved when the neurological exam and MRI of his brain came out negative. These are just a few of the purposeful measures I used with Neal. They are all included in one or more standard protocols. However, the prioritizing and timing of the introduction of each were unique to Neal's clinical situation.

Alan required that I catch on to the meaning a personal relationship with me had for him as a condition for his cooperating with both me and the other physicians treating his myelodysplasia.

Solomon was harder to read. In his case cooperation among his immunologist, internist, and myself (SAF) was efficient. It was his fear of pain and physical deterioration, hidden by stoicism, and his continual need to buck his son's and daughter-in-law's criticism, that made it so important to balance the attention I paid to his medical and personal complaints. His son insisted on slavish accountability from me, always questioning my judgment. He also consistently misread his father, accusing him of being "childish and lazy." Strategy in this situation necessitated that I assuage the son and daughter-in-law, while at the same time reassuring Solomon that his medical complaints were legitimate.

The personal and interpersonal factors at play in the clinical field

We apologize for complicating matters even further as we list the myriad factors that have a bearing on the clinical process. But, clinical work of any sort is indeed beset by complexities. At every moment the clinical field in both systemic medicine and psychiatry consists of the following.

Contributions to the clinical process

(1) Contributions from the patient.
   (a) The patient's part in facilitating the treatment.
   - His or her legitimate interest in receiving the physician's help.
   - His or her motivation to understand the disease, as well as capacity and desire to reflect on his or her own psychology as it effects the treatment.
   (b) The patient's contributions that confound this effort.
   - His or her needs and distortions as they color the clinical process.
   - His or her developmental and cultural limitations.
(2) Contributions from the physician.
   (a) Tools the physician uses to understand the patient.
   - His or her fund of information including theoretical beliefs, value system, and experience.
   - His or her particular capacity for understanding clinical events.
   - His or her personal *experience* of the patient's projections. Included is the patient partially recreating his or her own hope and despair within the physician through a psychological mechanism called "projective identification."[3]
   - The physician reacts personally to the patient; counter-transferences and reactions based in current reality included. When the patient responds in kind and the two are unaware of it, an interpersonally distorted interaction, an "enactment," results. Alan's internist's feeling that he was "sleazy" is an example.
   (b) Contributions from the physician that interfere with his or her ability to understand the patient: the physician contaminates treatment through his or her personality idiosyncrasies, theoretical biases, "blind spots," or inadvertent reactions.
(3) Non-verbal aspects of experience affecting the field in which treatment occurs.
   (a) The physician's supportive attitudes and actions.
   (b) Joint authorship: all experiences in treatment are shaped by both participants, physician and patient. Nothing belongs to either one alone. In these interactions the two may influence and change one another, at times in profound ways.

---

[3] Through this PI the physician's experience becomes analogous to that of the patient's. This exporting of experience occurs spontaneously, the recipient unaware it is occurring. Recognizing this is happening can dramatically improve a physician's understanding of a patient psychology and behavior. The "SO framework and analysis" described below provides a convenient vehicle for achieving this level of interpersonal appreciation.

(4) Subjectivity (Leder, 1990; Aron, 1996; Sullivan, 2003): subjectivity accounts for the absolute limitations in the physician's and patient's ability to understand each other. It imposes a fundamental restriction on what can be known at the moment by each. Because of the subjectivity of each one's experience, physician and patient are constantly compelled to depend on one another for information and feedback. Treatments are therefore, of necessity, collaborative undertakings. The subjectivity and inter-subjectivity (Orange *et al.*, 1997) of the participants' experiences is central in explaining why collaboration is so indispensable to their work.

Physician self-discipline: the Self-Other Rapid Assessment Method

Now to ways physicians can police themselves while engaged in the complicated matrix of diagnostic and treatment choices. The previously mentioned *Self-Other Rapid Assessment Framework* (SO framework), and the related treatment monitoring technique, *the Self-Other* (SO) *Rapid Assessment Method* (or, briefly, *the SO method*, or, equivalently, *the SO analysis*), offers a convenient, uncomplicated way for clinicians to keep track of their work. It represents a device for remaining in touch with the patient's current psychology and reactions to his or her systemic medical–psychiatric condition, as well as for the physician to keep track of his or her personal supporting or distorting contributions to that clinical situation.

The SO Rapid Assessment Method is based on a clinical construct, *the Self-Other* (SO) *Relational Configuration* (Frankel, S., 2007; Frankel, S., 2008), that incorporates a combined picture of the physician's and patient's internal and experiential life. Broken down, the structure of this model is as follows.

(1) At each clinical moment there are always at least two simultaneous sets of SO configurations at work for each person, one representing the physician's experience and one the patient's.

(2) Each person's SO configurations can be broken down into at least three subcategories: "self," "other", and "self with other." The "self with other" subcategory applies to the interaction between the two participants, in our case, the physician and patient.

(3) The product of the named three subcategories interfacing with one another constitutes a fourth SO category we have called "composite."

(4) As experienced, each set of SO configurations, one belonging to the physician and the other to the patient, contributes to creating the state of mind of each treatment participant.

At any given moment in treatment there is usually more than one set of SOs (SO configurations) in play in the clinical field; often several different SO sets associated with each participant. For example, a patient can be simultaneously angry at and appreciative toward her physician, each attitude having separate clinical influence. The value of a physician keeping an inventory of current SOs is obvious in psychiatry, the complexity of the patient's experiences inherently of interest to psychiatrists. In other areas of medicine SO readings can, however, be equally useful for tracking how well the patient understands and can comply with treatment.

We are adding the following for the sake of completeness in understanding the SO concept (Frankel, S., 1995, pp. 150–152).

(a) The personal and interpersonal field in treatment generally consists of multiple, often conflicting, SO configurations.

(b) Each SO configuration may link with current or past experiences outside of the physician–patient relationship; for example, one centered on an abusive relationship with a parent and predisposing the patient to feel victimized.

(c) Some SOs are primarily initiated by and carried on by one treatment partner; others are partially or fully introduced by and shared between the partners.

(d) An SO analysis can also be made more accurate by incorporating in it innate personality features such as intelligence or personality traits.

Clinical illustrations involving conflicting SOs

Stop. Help. What does all this have to do with general medicine?

Think of Alan. Who was he, a willing patient, or a rebel who couldn't be trusted? Obviously he was both at the same time. You can use this dichotomy to construct two different SOs, each describing an aspect of Alan's character. Neither SO alone, however, would fully capture who Alan was. Understanding both would have been helpful for his optimal clinical management.

The parallel in psychiatry is familiar. Lucy, a 57-year-old mother of three, remained committed to working with me (SAF) even as she became frustrated with what she believed was my disinterest in providing practical guidance in her struggle to help her children. She was originally referred to me by her primary care provider when that physician found it difficult to deal with Lucy's global anxiety and her multiple, vague somatic complaints. Lucy had been separated from her family during the Holocaust and was constantly worried about the welfare of her grown children. While Lucy's trust of me existed independently of her impatience, it also protected her against recognizing her frustration with me and concern about alienating me. Her friendliness in treatment served a defensive and protective function.

The following is a brief summary of a dialogue between Lucy and me. As Lucy spoke about her son struggling to repair a fated relationship with a woman, she remembered her childhood desperation when her father had to leave Poland for Russia to work for three years. Simultaneously, my vacation was approaching. She switched the topic from her son to this memory, saying she felt a sense of hopelessness in connection with my leaving; yet I was "still there being pleasant and supportive." She had a hard time understanding the juxtaposition of these two states of mind. However, since Lucy's mother always encouraged forbearance, she appealed to that memory. At such moments, Lucy said, it was as if her mother were exhorting her to be strong. My style was different from her mother's, who had been lost in tragedy and resigned to stoicism during most of Lucy's early life. With me, because I believed her son might be able to have a successful relationship with a woman, Lucy could imagine success as a mother.

In this example, Lucy was of two, almost equally balanced states of mind (SOs). In one she saw only abandonment and despair. In the other, she implicitly trusted me, believing I would not let her down.

The relationship between clinical field complexity and clinical judgment

How can a physician work effectively if he or she has to think deliberately about each factor influencing a treatment? If a practitioner did that, the treatment he or she provided would certainly be halting, deprived of the spontaneity that goes with the effective application of clinical judgment.

Consider all the factors that come into play when driving a car. From moment to moment you usually don't think about whether you should steer a little more to the left or if you should touch the brake. Driving is usually more automatic than that.

While in the driver's seat, observe the idiosyncrasies of other drivers on the road and notice the extent to which you spontaneously correct for their habits. At the same time, note that you probably are thinking consciously about your destination and making deliberate corrections when your safety is at risk.

Return to clinical judgment and the strategies we adopt when dealing with patients. While the thought may not be entirely comforting, to a significant extent many clinical decisions are semi-automatic. Imagine deliberately thinking out each move in clinical work and picture how ineffective you would become if you did that.

How to use the SO framework in the context of clinical complexity

We are advocating the use of the SO framework for physicians as they make decisions about treatment interventions, especially as clinical requirements shift. There are other convenient methods of physician self-assessment, for example Casement's (1985) self-supervision method, a technique that is used mainly in psychotherapy. However, in comparison to the SO method, these techniques tend to be restricted in their scope or versatility and therefore are of limited usefulness for physicians and other medical professionals who need to make rapid and incisive assessments. Examples of the use of the SO method to check and direct the work with Solomon and Neal follow.

Solomon

Solomon was ostensibly cooperative with treatment. He was sharp and motivated. The difficulty was that, when it came to applying the recommendations of his physicians, he incessantly dragged his feet. It was a challenge to identify the unspoken factors creating this dissidence and the extent to which they would continue to create havoc with treatment.

Interestingly, the SO method, as applied to his treatment at this point, uncovered depths of fear and discouragement (the "self" component) as well as distrust of others' capacity to understand his needs (the "other" component). On the "self with other" side, he had withdrawn sharply and there was little chance that he could – or given his deteriorating medical condition, even should – become interested in taking a hopeful stance about his future. A good argument could be made for his actually being content with his now quite empty life and the validity of his claim that he was privately preparing to die; a stance requiring him to resist both his family's and his physicians' forceful agendas.

Neal

Neal tells me about Renee, a new girl in his life. "She's OK, really cute and sexy, but young. I did spend the last two days with her. But, really she's not so great." He then added with a gleam in his eye, "But, we do have plans for this weekend."

Confusing? It certainly was for me (SAF) at first. And, I was concerned about how quickly Neal could get involved and recalled how hard he fell, at times to a point verging on suicide, when women became tired of him. And, that seemed to have happened a lot in the past.

What to do in Neal's treatment at that moment? How could I tell? I had several choices. I could inquire further about his infatuation and express pleasure about his having a new romance. I could tell him about my concerns and remind him of his history of failed involvements and the disastrous impact each had on his earlier life. I could also have considered mentioning Renee to his parents, asking them to watch carefully and report any worrisome change in Neal's moods. Apart from using my intuition, which was that I should sound the alarm to Neal and possibly even to his parents, how was I to decide?

Enter the SO analysis. Let's try it on for size.

(1) Begin with the "self" dimension. Neal told me that he lacked confidence in his relationships with women. If a woman paid attention to him he was flattered. On this dimension, Renee apparently had hooked Neal. It was when being flattered turned sour that the worry I was having was likely to become relevant. At these times the potential for a crash in Neal's self-esteem always threatened to create havoc. That is what happened in college when Dorothy let him down and Neal saturated himself with alcohol and drove his car wildly in front of a police station screaming insults at the police.

(2) On the "other" dimension, notice that Neal knew very little about Renee except that she was sexy and younger than him.

(3) Moving to the "self with other" dimension, there was little evidence of a heartfelt connection between Renee and Neal. And, here was the problem. Neal privately had big plans for being with Renee in spite of the fact that he hardly knew her. He actually had little reason to have confidence that she would maintain a relationship with him.

Added up, the situation, when subjected to an SO analysis, read out as worrisome, with Neal potentially setting himself up for another personal catastrophe. To understand Neal, it was necessary to factor in his 22-year-old developmental status and the ease with which he could feel personally devastated. The SO analysis supported my intuition about what to do clinically, its use adding a deliberate, orienting step to the decision-making process.

The results were as follows.

(1) The logic, based on Neal's history, appeared to be that Neal could become dangerously over-invested in a relationship after knowing too little about the person with whom he was becoming involved. According to the SO analysis, that could be happening in this situation.

(2) The implication, as I (SAF) understood it, was to warn Neal, but be careful not to humiliate him. And, that is what I did.

Close inspection of the state of mind I am calling "intuition" would reveal that my choosing to warn Neal was at least partially the product of years of clinical experience aided by a reasoning process with both deliberate and automatic aspects. Under this microscope, the "intuition" I used in this case begins, then, to look increasingly like what we call "clinical judgment" or, in this case, "experi-ence-based clinical judgment (EBCJ)" connoting a semi-deliberate, stepwise cognitive sequence.

Turning again to the reality of practice, how does one do repeated SO analyses in those demanding situations and not get bogged down in obsessive detail? How inconvenient is it for a physician, psychiatrist or not, to carry out these procedures? Our suggestion is that you try it. Using SO analyses is actually rather simple and may well introduce another valuable truing device into your work. The SO framework can be employed regularly or at points of urgency. It has the potential of reminding you of the interpersonal complexity of the systemic medical or psychiatric situation you are managing and of providing a useful way to negotiate it.

The use of the SO analysis by the MPCP

How does all this discussion about the SO analysis apply to the MPCP in his or her coordinating role? After all, many of our truing devices are tools for individual practitioners working on the front lines. First, it is a great advantage for the MPCP, in addition to the individual team members, to use the *SO Rapid Assessment Method* to check his or her impressions of the patient. Second, it is the MPCP's job to evaluate the rigor of each team member's work, keeping an eye on whether that person is consistently using truing measures appropriate to his or her specialty. Finally, the MPCP is responsible for collaboratively updating and following outcome criteria. This process utilizes test data and ratings of treatment progress which ideally include clinical determinations of the patient's status.

Intuition and clinical judgment in the choices physicians make

Physicians are constantly making choices, an abundance of small ones and others that are bigger, while negotiating the complexity of clinical problems. These decisions are for the most part not articulated. They are guided by factors inherent in what we are calling "clinical judgment," once again a step beyond "intuition." If we study the outcome of these sequences we might be impressed by how often they are on target, even though the steps in arriving at them may be obscure (see the argument for the major place of "contextual," non-specific, factors in creating clinical change, e.g., Frank & Frank, 1991; Wampold, 2001; Norcross, 2002; Hill & Lambert, 2004; Novotny & Thompson-Brenner, 2004). But, now add physician monitoring in the form of repeat laboratory, diagnostic imaging, or psychometric assessment, as well as intermittent SO analyses, and the clinical process truly begins to cohere.

For "operationally complex" treatments insert an MPCP, his or her coordinating role, as well as unique personal and clinical impact on the patient. On the personal side, he or she delivers a category of objectivity and leadership different from that provided by any other team member. In making this statement we are not referring to the MPCP in a direct service role, but more particularly to the MPCP's careful monitoring of the patient's overriding treatment goals, the work of making sure treatment always moves in the direction of satisfying outcome goals.

What about clinical experience? How much does it really matter for insuring the effectiveness of what an individual physician and MPCP do? Logically, length and depth of experience tend to be correlated with improved outcome.

The learning curve flattens out after a while, however (Ritter & Schooler, 2001; Reichenbach et al., 2006). After doing a certain number of a particular kind of operation or seeing numerous depressed patients, a physician has a reasonably clear idea of how to do that procedure or manage that clinical problem. But, even here we need to beware, since agreement among seasoned clinicians is never perfect and sometimes the accuracy of their clinical assessments is not much better than those who are less experienced (Robinson et al., 1999; Grantcharov et al., 2002). Here of course, again, is the ever-present argument for the use of truing devices, the monitoring referred to above, to negotiate clinical complexity.

Think of the complexity of the cases we have discussed. None, not Alan, Neal, Keith, nor Solomon, had difficulties that conformed to a single, straightforward systemic medical or psychiatric diagnosis. Physicians, along with all other clinicians, always work in a complex practice field infused with subjectivity, and consistently need to identify ways to improve their clinical accuracy. Much of what we do involves clinical judgment. And, there is rarely a situation in which our choices cannot be improved though the use of clinically appropriate truing devices.

6

The intersection of data and clinical judgment: the place of subjectivity in treatment decisions

We celebrate the accountability and increased objectivity that evidence-based medicine (EBM) and empirically supported treatment (EST) have brought to our work. However, it seems counterintuitive, in conflict with the role judgment plays in all clinical work, to overlook the personal factors and technical controversies that complicate almost all medical treatments. There is every argument for following an evidence-based protocol created for a particular diagnosis. Use it as you formulate and follow a treatment plan. Beware, however, of overlooking the fact that the diagnoses on which evidence-based and empirically supported treatments are predicated are prototype approximations of what the physician is likely to encounter in the office (Westen *et al.*, 2002; Weinberger & Westen, 2004).

There is rarely a situation in medicine that is not "muddied" by technical controversy; for example, about the best way to manage bone marrow failure such as Alan's. Added, are the personal and cultural considerations unique to each patient and influencing his or her compliance with treatment. And then there are the co-morbidities, coexisting and overlapping diagnostic entities, that complicate diagnosis and treatment planning. For example, as with Alan, do you chance a bone marrow transplant for a patient with significant splenomegaly or a current cytomegalovirus infection outbreak? Alan was afflicted with both. What steps do you take to make that judgment? Are you willing to take the risks involved? Is the patient?

Similarly, psychiatric diagnosis in real-life situations is rarely clear-cut. Millon (1996) makes the critical point that a specific diagnosis of psychopathology frequently has a personality disorder component associated with it, influencing treatment selection and skewing prognosis.

Given the multiple contaminating and enhancing technical considerations, as well as unique agendas, the illness, the physician, and the patient each introduce into treatment, we come back to the question of how do physician and patient accurately find their way toward the most effective treatment interventions?

The physician needs to act

Here, then, is the practical dilemma. As physicians we need to be rigorous about our work. Few clinical factors can be overlooked. However, if we get too lost in clinical complexity, we run the risk of bogging down the process. Physicians need to act. They have a finite amount of time to make decisions.

Our response to the question about finding one's way, then, is the following:
(1) First, to underscore the fact that clinical work is rarely straightforward, without technical and interpersonal challenges.
(2) Second, to acknowledge that, more often than not, the physician and patient do seem to stay on course. In part, and often in large part, the physician's contribution involves the use of *experience-based clinical judgment* (EBCJ), a state of mind nonetheless encumbered with subjectivity.
(3) Third, if the physician did not work in this way and was unable to employ sound clinical judgment for guidance, he or she would run the risk of becoming handicapped by a plethora of clinical details.

In short, because of the need to be decisive and exercise clinical judgment when on the firing line, some precision may have to be sacrificed to exigency. Our solution to this dilemma, the pull between precision and pace, is to find and invoke truing devices that can be used conveniently to improve treatment accuracy.

Truing methods in this category include the physician self-monitoring described in Chapter 5, in particular the *SO (Self-Other) Rapid Assessment Method*, as well as brief psychometric protocols and symptom check lists. Laboratory tests and diagnostic imaging are mentioned in Chapter 3. Other guides, listed in Chapter 2, include personal, school, and work history. These, as well as information from collateral sources, are easy to get and can provide a sense for how well the patient can commit to treatment. Another example is the use of trial periods of treatment strategy followed by shared and collaboratively modified treatment plans for the purpose of improving clinical accuracy and engaging the patient as an ally.

In this vein, we note that one of the most convenient devices to sharpen clinical work is frank discussions between patient and physician. Ironically, this truing device, collaboration about treatment progress and goals between physician and patient, is often underestimated and not pursued deliberately.

Physician–patient collaboration and its impact on physician judgment

Related to the topic of physician–patient collaboration is the previously mentioned issue of physician–patient reciprocity. Respectful dialogue between physician and patient, with the patient influencing the physician's decisions, is an essential component of successful treatment.

Solomon made no bones about this issue. The more his son insisted he observe better hygiene, bathe, and have the lesions on his body debrided regularly, the more this otherwise clear-thinking man resisted. Having the scabs removed was painful and discouraging to him. In the process, he had to view his deteriorating body and it repulsed him, always reminding him of the progression of his disease. But, most particularly, he did not like his son and daughter-in-law's authoritarian manner. Eventually he became entrenched in his resistance to it, claiming with growing disingenuousness that he was following their orders. By that time all he cared about was getting them off his back. While ordinarily a good collaborator in treatment, under his family's unrelenting surveillance Solomon shut down. Going back to clinical judgment, I (SAF) reasoned that Solomon would most likely cooperate if they eased up, and I repeatedly told them that; making sure I did not push him either. Sadly, they never relented, and, ironically, it was a septicemia originating in his festering lesions that was ultimately responsible for his death.

Return to Neal. At this point we will bypass a description of the workups by medical specialists, which Neal required to assess his attentional difficulties, headaches, neck and back pain, and visual symptoms, in favor of highlighting the clinical judgment and candidness required for managing his psychiatric needs.

Neal told me that his father was "crazy." Since I (SAF) knew both Neal and his father, I was not surprised by that kind of comment from Neal, and, at the same time, I found myself more than a little skeptical about its accuracy. Neal's father had never seemed even a little bit deranged to me. So, what should I have said to Neal? It would have been dishonest for me to take a "customer is always right" stance with him. What, in fact, I decided to do – my clinical judgment – was to take his perception as a possibility and wrap my mind around the idea. That way I would be able to mine any truth out of Neal's opinion of his father and do the least damage to our rapport. To what behaviors of his father could Neal be referring? When did they occur? Could Neal entertain the possibility that his verdict might be colored by his need to disenfranchise his father in order to emancipate himself? How to maintain my goal of supporting Neal and the treatment, and remain appropriately strategic and objective at the same time?

Both Solomon and Neal also illustrate one of the major asymmetries inherent in all treatments: the judgment required to support the physician's leading role in creating and implementing treatment strategies. As discussed in Chapter 5, the clinical process is inherently asymmetrical, with the treating physician regularly in the lead.

Solomon made it clear that I needed to regulate my probing about his attitude toward his personal hygiene while he was chafing under his son's and daughter-in-law's tyranny. I was certain that he was doing himself a disservice medically by allowing his infected lesions to fulminate. Once clear of family pressure, I discerned that we would be able to take this medical issue on more directly. I was in the role of managing the treatment, and my decision about this matter needed to be a strategic one.

I found myself paradoxically acting more gingerly with Neal as he made his seemingly absurd judgments of his father. His non-verbal message to me was that he would be put off if I confronted him with my opinion about the distorted nature of his allegation. In spite of my liaison with his parents at that time, I instinctively decided to keep information about Neal's attitude to myself, reasoning that if I told his parents I would both be betraying Neal and could lose the father's close cooperation. I depended heavily on the parents' support during this period. This was the judgment I used and the clinical strategy I decided upon for that moment.

In a well-functioning treatment, the balance between the physician's and patient's authority is repeatedly shifted toward greater parity, each party having moments of greater influence. Solomon's taking the lead in determining when he would be ready for me to be more instructional about his hygiene is a good example. Our impression is that this trading of influence occurs in all treatments, whether or not it is acknowledged.

From our point of view, the most successful treatments in medicine are collaborative (Frankel, R. *et al.*, 2003; Charon, 2006; Frankel, R. & Inui, 2006; Frankel, S., 2007). The physician and patient join forces persistently; at points effecting an equivalence of authority and wisdom, at other times locating impetus for this joining in the other.

Little needs to be said at this point about how the role of the MPCP fits with these principles. The MPCP is the hub of an intricate network of collaborations. These interactions allow the MPCP to sequence and prioritize treatment interventions. Keith's story, below, is a good example of what can happen when this process fails.

Using multiple truing measures to support clinical judgment

Any experienced physician will tell you that, frequently, the most important source of data in a psychiatric or systemic medical assessment is clinical – what you see and hear from and about the patient. Happily this point of view fits with the idea that clinical judgment used by a seasoned physician is often close to the mark. But, how reliable is this subjectively infused source of information for physician guidance, especially when placed against the test-based assessments described in Chapter 3? Of course, the answer is that the accuracy of the clinical process improves, often incrementally, as more sources of data are introduced (Henderson & Keiding, 2005).

The argument here is for the simultaneous and successive use of truing devices, in concert with clinical judgment. Supporting this statement is the fact that requirements in treatment change regularly. It is worth noting that this observation limits the usefulness of ESTs and EBTs, since they specify fixed criteria for working with each type or cluster of illnesses. The physician and patient as treatment partners, and particularly the physician in his or her leadership role, need to be vigilant about and accommodate to these shifts, with the physician using all available truing devices together with clinical judgment to stay on track.

Move now to the world of the MPCP, the multiple sources of data available to that person, and the proper place of clinical judgment in that work. He or she needs to make sure communication is maintained with all team members and that each one's work reflects acceptable clinical standards.

As MPCP I (SAF) needed to be certain, for example, that Solomon's internist was aware of the extent to which Solomon neglected his hygiene and the likelihood that his TPN shunt could become infected as a result. The internist had to be counseled about how to communicate with and not just lecture Solomon about this issue. To this end, I accompanied Solomon to several of his appointments at the internist's office with the objective of judiciously introducing this topic into their conversation. I also needed to prompt Solomon's immunologist to set a regular schedule for forwarding progress notes and laboratory reports to the other physicians involved in his care. The immunologist had been remiss about these communications, presumably because of Solomon's passivity about maintaining contact with him. Then, there was the conflict between Solomon and his family members as it affected his compliance with medical treatment. Taking this matter in hand, I talked with Solomon's son and daughter-in-law on a biweekly basis.

Putting it together: Keith, a case of failed clinical judgment

From the point of view of medical management, at age 73, Keith's experience as his polycythemia vera reached an end stage was distinctly more troubling than Alan's. This difference was ironic since Alan's myelofibrosis had progressed much more quickly and was more debilitating than Keith's illness. Both men had a hematological illness. The issues involved in medical management of Keith's polycythemia vera and Alan's progressive myelofibrosis were similar once the diseases had advanced. Myelofibrosis almost always moves more quickly than polycythemia vera, leading to death in about five years, but both eventuate in the failure of multiple organ systems as conversion to leukemia occurs.

While Alan sought and received excellent medical care, it was he who introduced the main distortions in communication with his physicians. Keith, on the other hand, was blindsided by an over-zealous internist. This physician had also been a golf partner of his and, as a result of this extra-clinical relationship, he took a "proprietary" interest in what he believed was Keith's welfare.

My (SAF) role with Keith was at first incidental. I had been his wife's psychiatrist and had helped them when their problems as a couple became hard to manage. Keith grew to respect me, finding the work I did helpful. When his polycythemia vera entered its final stage, he asked to meet with me to help him prepare for his impending death. Keith was a private person, strong throughout his life, not the least bit psychologically minded. He said he was determined to accomplish this final episode as well as he had done everything else in his life.

Ironically, the person who could not accept Keith's prognosis and wish for dignity during this final episode was his internist. Dr. R. had been approached repeatedly by both myself and Keith's wife to collaborate. However, while he was civil in his communications with us, he seemed interested in little more than patient compliance and medical authority over the other physicians involved in the case. His singular agenda was to keep Keith alive, and he insisted on increasingly heroic and disabling medical measures to do so. When any of us objected to his choices, he further limited his communication with us. In short, truing measures in this clinical situation were selected and controlled by a single person, the primary care physician, who relied exclusively on the measures he selected and his own judgment to provide direction for the treatment.

The internist's decisions ultimately required that Keith be hospitalized for months at a time at a location distant from Keith's home and the convalescent facility nearby. Medically, these treatments did indeed slow Keith's demise, perhaps by a year or two. But for what? As a complication of Keith's progressing medical condition and its treatment, he also developed dementia secondary to thrombotic microangiopathy. His wife and I begged the internist to stop his heroics and let Keith die comfortably, but his response was to become even more insistent on his authority and, as before, less communicative.

Poor Keith. He was deprived of his considerable pride and emphatic wish to maintain control of his personal life during his last months. His decline and eventual death – a year or two after he said a dignified good-bye to his four children – were hideous. Had his internist been more willing to work collaboratively with Keith, his wife, myself, and other physicians, respecting Keith's original desire to die before he lost all sense of dignity, the final course and outcome of treatment would likely have been quite different. In this case, one physician's clinical judgment, my own, was subverted by another's, and the other physician was absolutely fixed in his decision not to be collaborative.

And, the moral of this story? The MPCP's role needs to be formalized at the beginning of a team-based treatment. Subversion of the collaborative model, with the judgment and influence of physician overshadowing all else as it did in Keith's case, needs to be handled according to "the established laws" governing that team's collective behavior. There should be a proper "investigation," the MPCP amassing the facts, and then a meeting where the MPCP and the dissident team member, or in some cases the entire team, meet to consider the dissatisfied member's position. The resulting consensus then needs to be shared, discussed by team members, and incorporated into a revised treatment plan.

Neal, clinical judgment that succeeded

Bright, creative, maybe brilliant. Irascible and unfocused. Painfully shy and yet socially ambitious. I assume these are enough contradictions to drive any parent, friend, or even physician, to distraction. As you will recall, it was Neal's father who was supposed to be off-balance. But, could it have been Neal who "drove him crazy"?

Confusing? An interesting clinical challenge? But, mainly the work with Neal at this point was personally trying for me (SAF), and I am surprised that I sustained my commitment so faithfully. Recall that we are excluding from this description the several possible systemic medical concerns troubling Neal.

For the first six months Neal was simply a captive audience. Clearly, his life was failing. He could not settle down, attend school, and he drank too much: all significant concerns for those involved in his life. But, in his mind, the treatment was foisted on him and he had grave doubts about whether he needed it. He did see himself as faltering, but was oddly resistant to getting any help. He wasn't arrogant, just edgy; always restless. For me, simply holding Neal "still" was challenging. Yet, he was about ready to sink if he didn't commit to some kind of treatment. There were plenty of decisions for me to make during this period; each requiring clinical judgment, and each needing to be formulated on the spot.

So far, there were at least three personal agendas at issue outside of Neal's psychiatric and systemic medical concerns, each influencing the course of the treatment and each impacting me as the treating psychiatrist and treatment coordinator. They included: (1) Neal's parents' desire to have their son "cured," (2) Neal's pressing interest in rejoining his friends from the university he had to leave earlier that year, and (3) my desire to provide good patient care. It was not just our agendas that impacted my judgment and strategic decisions as treatment coordinator, but also how we each understood the situation. Neal's parents saw him as deliberately "mean" and irreparably "damaged," while Neal saw them as insufferably stupid. We have summarized the bare bones of the "self," "other," and "self with other" dimensions of this case in Chapter 4.

Regarding the ultimate course of this treatment, I have to make a confession. I really do not know what I did that mattered to Neal in the beginning of our work other than my seizing on his parents' conviction that their son needed help and that something had to be done. So, at first I was mainly persistent. I hung on for dear life, no matter how much or how often the uninitiated Neal tried to shake me off. I doubt that at that point Neal saw me as anything more than an irritating presence who should have no place in his life.

On the other hand, Neal was smart and curious, so he ultimately acceded to a neuropsychological assessment. He was also worried about the possibility that he had sustained brain damage from his overuse of alcohol and other substances, and was glad to be referred to a neurologist at that point. We were helped to maintain our course when both the neuropsychologist and neurologist, at my suggestion, insisted with Neal that he was substantially affected by ADHD, needed a stimulant medication, and could use help in learning how to settle down, instead of frenetically moving from relationship to relationship and project to project. Following this intervention, Neal even agreed to enroll in a CBT psychoeducational and treatment series targeted to address his ADHD. Note, how often my clinical judgment was called for in this clinical sequence; judgments that were informed by intuition and clinical experience, but also by test-based data and collaboration with collateral sources including another physician.

And, things began to change. Neal slowed down long enough to apply for several computer programming jobs, and got each one. The ne'er do well was inching his way toward success.

Imperceptibly, gradually, Neal's attitude toward me began to shift. Lo and behold, over weeks he started to talk, providing evidence that my strategy was working. Though still grumpy and not very conversational, Neal was beginning to take my advice and started to welcome coming to see me. I infer that, apart from the effects of the dextroamphetamine–amphetamine combination he was taking, this change reflected the fact that he was now seeing results. He had something to look forward to. And then, out of the blue, the big announcement. "You know, Steve, I don't really look forward to it, but I think if I'm going to have any future I'd better go back to school." It was as quick and non-dramatic as that. And, he did it. He returned to school and has been successful academically and personally, with the added help of only occasional telephone appointments with me.

The components

There were three clinical truing mechanisms, in addition to experience-based clinical judgments (EBCJs), that were particularly useful in keeping on track with Neal and Keith. Each obviously contributed to my conviction about how to act with the patient.

These are listed here.

(1) I took frequent SO readings. At first this measure helped me establish where Neal stood in his ability to work in treatment and then to follow him as we witnessed improvement in his self-esteem and capability with relationships. With Keith, the SO method helped expose how his sense of agency was being undermined by his physician, making it hard for him to think and act on his own.

(2) Added, is collaboration between the physician and the patient. Neal and I constantly assessed his attitude toward treatment, the possibility of returning to school, and his parents. Keith and I fell successively "out of synch" as Dr. R. stopped communicating with me.

(3) Finally, there were formal assessment methods. In Neal's case the neuropsychological assessment confirmed my suspicion that, in spite of his

discouragement and negativity, he was psychiatrically healthier than his parents believed. In Keith's case, the evolving course of his leukemia, paired with a neuropsychological assessment, confirmed the diagnosis of dementia, and made everyone but his internist skeptical about the wisdom of prolonging his life.

How much more accurate are we likely to be in our work when we incorporate these three truing mechanisms? This is not a trivial question, and the response is a bit convoluted. The answer – perhaps frustrating for those of us who require categorical guidelines – is specific to each clinical process. The physician, not the statistician, needs to ascertain whether each truing mechanism contributes incremental validity to the particular diagnostic and treatment procedure at hand. The "incremental validity" of a truing sequence builds as each new truing mechanism adds to the data other truing mechanisms have already provided.

To the extent that each truing mechanism adds specificity to the mix, accuracy is increased. If it doesn't, then bringing in more information through the same method(s) is redundant: a waste of time. If you are certain your patient suffers from diabetes mellitus or is overly anxious, the truing devices you need are not those that verify the presence or absence of diabetes mellitus or an anxiety disorder. Instead you need diagnostic procedures that give additional information about the patient's particular affliction, its more subtle aspects.

Outcome measures

Finally, to judge the effectiveness of a clinical process we move to the ultimate criteria for success: results (McGrady et al., 1995; Hill & Lambert, 2004; Bickman, 2008; Haywood et al., 2012). It really doesn't matter what you do technically to make a case work if you do not get results. Tracking and confirming results by identifying and formally following outcome measures provides a way to confirm or override clinical judgment. In primary care medicine, outcome criteria usually conform to problem areas identified by medical tests and diagnostic imaging procedures, although subjective reports of patient status count as well. In psychiatry, outcome measures are generally delineated through conversation with the patient or psychometric assessment. SO determinations and psychometric measures can be used for outcome determination in both specialties.

Move again to complex cases where following outcome is in the purview of an MPCP. While each team member tracks progress in his or her specialty area, the MPCP is accountable for the overall success of the case. When movement has stopped, the MPCP has the responsibility of alerting team members and, in collaboration with them, effecting a change in the treatment plan.

The place of clinical judgment in creating and implementing strategy

There are, yet, additional considerations when implementing clinical strategy, and again clinical judgment becomes the ultimate determinant for how to proceed. For example, what to do about revealing one's clinical strategy to a patient? You simply have to be judicious about what you divulge. In treatment you frequently do not say everything about your strategy at every juncture. Keith would almost certainly have objected to hearing my (SAF) uncensored opinion about his internist. He was afraid not to be grateful to the physician who in fact was orchestrating a treatment hostile to his desires. I needed other ways to counter that physician's uncomprehending influence. To the best of my ability I did that directly through regular conversations with Keith's wife and indirectly by frequently visiting Keith at the hospital. As a second example, I am sure that had I revealed my strategy to Neal early in our work he would have bolted. Full disclosure at each point in a treatment with someone like Neal is about as useful to productive coexistence as soliciting your teenager's approval for each rule you set down.

As was stated in Chapter 5, strategic thinking is ubiquitous in clinical work, whether acknowledged or not (Chan *et al.*, 2001; Fava *et al.*, 2011). At the same time, given its partially subjective nature, we still need to remain skeptical about being too dependent on it. In searching for an antidote to this dilemma, however, it may be tempting to fall back too heavily on evidence-based treatment protocols and the apparent objectivity they offer.

Here's the hitch. As we work our way through a treatment, we never can escape imprecision, or, when we seem to get it right, the problem often becomes not exactly knowing how that happened. "Clinical judgment" is used by seasoned physicians as a comforting phrase, at times suggesting that the physician knows just what he or she is doing. Empirically supported treatments (ESTs) and evidence-based treatments (EBTs) are quite specific, but often provide a false sense of security. Indeed, truing helps, especially if carried out deliberately. But, when all is said and done, you still have a massive amount of unmapped territory to negotiate with any patient, and much of the negotiation may occur spontaneously, fueled by intuition that leads to judgment calls that are often – when backed by experience – reasonably accurate.

In the next chapter we again take on the subject of clinical strategy; this time asking the question of how it is formulated and implemented with accuracy.

7

Clinical strategy: grappling with treatment complexity

It's true. Invoking strategy, its technical and especially its interpersonal aspects, can be understood as problematic when it comes to clinical work. Strategy may imply coercion, potentially putting the physician, whether psychiatrist or PCP, in a position of unjustified authority (Greenberg, 1986, 1999; Hoffman, 1996; Mitchell, 1997) and compromising what is otherwise supposed to be a relatively dispassionate professional stance. We were originally going to restrict our definition of clinical strategy to its technical aspects. While indeed strategy is and should be based on technical considerations, what then happens to the more subjective interpersonal aspects, the patient–physician relationship and the treatment alliance? Contemporary research in both psychiatry and primary care medicine underscores the central place that the treatment relationship plays in outcome (Frank & Frank, 1991; Najavits & Strupp, 1994; Krupnick *et al.*, 1996; Barber *et al.*, 2000; Roter, 2000; Wampold, 2001; Frankel, R., 2004; Norcross *et al.*, 2006; Hilsenroth & Cromer, 2007).

Solomon and I (SAF) admired Solomon's internist. He was a superb physician, but he repeatedly had bad news for Solomon: news Solomon didn't want to hear. Fortunately, unlike Keith's ambitious internist, he was not "proprietary." He realized that without Solomon's heartfelt cooperation the treatment he offered would be impossibly handicapped. Solomon would sit endlessly in his apartment watching cooking shows on TV, moping while he stared at gourmet dishes he would never again be able to eat because of the toll his scleroderma had already taken on his esophagus and stomach. The internist liked Solomon and took his role quite seriously but hardly had the time to work with Solomon's depression and emotional inaccessibility.

As I took over as Solomon's MPCP I did need to find that time, however. My role was to pay close attention to his entire clinical situation, making sure his basic needs were being met. Since Solomon had been missing medical appointments, the strategy the internist and I developed included my holding some treatment sessions at Solomon's apartment, Martha Stewart blaring in the background. Also, if you recall, Solomon's mobility was limited because of severe arthritis affecting both replaced hips, and he understood my willingness to come to him as an appropriate response to his disability. As well, we decided that I would occasionally accompany Solomon to his medical appointments since his complicated care had become disorganized. On one occasion, also, Solomon invited me to join him at his retirement facility for lunch. It was "an eye-opener," since, by comparing Solomon with other elderly residents, I could judge the extent of Solomon's lethargy and discouragement. It also provided me with a view of Solomon's restricted interactions with others.

Solomon's internist and I talked and emailed regularly. According to our plan, I took responsibility for engaging and following through with the many medical specialists Solomon had heretofore been avoiding. Soon, there was an immunologist, a dermatologist, a gastroenterologist, and a pulmonologist on board. My taking over this coordinating function was urgent, since the secret Solomon was guarding from friends and family had mainly to do with his perceptive assessment of his seriously deteriorating health.

And Keith? The only interpersonal strategy his internist used was to chat about their past golf relationship and then intimidate him with claimed medical consequences if Keith didn't comply with his progressively draconian regimen. Rather than collaborate with other physicians like myself, he insisted on doing almost everything by himself. And, perhaps most damaging, he forcefully excluded Keith's wife from involvement in decisions affecting Keith's welfare. Instead, Keith's physician generally announced changes in treatment plans after they had been instituted medically, making it impossible for any of us to react to them in a timely and effective way. Our wishes, just like Keith's, apparently didn't very much count to him.

As we see it, the reason for strategy in clinical work is that the physician, or MPCP as leader of the treatment team in "operationally complex" cases, is ultimately responsible for outcome, for doing his or her part to facilitate the desired result. So, it makes perfect sense from a physician's point of view to map out the field in which the treatment is occurring and put the pieces together in a way that works; that is, strategically. If the physician does not do this deliberately, he or she is likely to do so automatically. Take these principles to the MPCP level and the place of strategy is even more obvious. Can you imagine an MPCP operating without a formal treatment plan that includes a strategy which is regularly revised as the ground rules for the treatment shift?

Added and not quantifiable in this process is the physician's earnestness: his or her heartfelt desire to be medically helpful and how this is communicated to the patient. Incidentally, patients benefit from earnestness too. Physicians respond well to that quality (Frankel, S., 2000).

Here are some of the imponderables. Each plays its part in how the physician and patient behave and therefore in their revealed or unstated strategies for engaging each other:

(1) unspoken agendas contributed individually by the physician and patient, including the personal biases, transferences, and countertransferences the patient and physician bring to bear as they work;

(2) the physician's and patient's personal limitations, many idiosyncratic and related to his or her background;

(3) cultural considerations influencing both the physician and patient;

(4) current events in each participant's life;

(5) biological influences on the physician's and patient's state of mind;

(6) the personal and formal theories the physician and patient hold about how change occurs thorough interpersonal influence in treatment.

Adding to the above influences on how a physician thinks and conducts him or herself in treatment are the components of the treatment field listed in Chapter 6. Each named factor needs to be taken into account in terms of the way it affects and gives direction to therapeutic movement. However, much of this activity occurs silently. Clinical truing devices such as repeat interviews, examinations, and laboratory tests, SO analyses, and patient–physician collaboration all contribute to making the strategic process more comprehensible and deliberate.

Again, moving to the level of the MPCP, that person needs to take into consideration – deal with and integrate into the treatment plan – all factors impinging on the patient as well as on each member of the treatment team. The psychologies at issue are those of the individual team members and the team members interacting. Sound like a hectic job? Well, it is! Doing this work well is complicated, with the immunologist's findings in the foreground at the beginning of this week, a new symptom suddenly coming up a few days later and mandating that the MPCP confer with team members, and the insurance company balking about a critical procedure and throwing the patient's family into a panic at the start of the next week.

Subjectivity creates more complexity

To illustrate the way details can escape us unless we deliberately set out to appreciate them, let us turn our attention to a new metaphor: cliff scaling. El Capitan is a magnificent rock face gazing down on visitors to Yosemite Valley in California. Its regal blues, greens, and grays mingle, shifting playfully as the sun moves across its horizon.

An illusion? No and yes. From the valley, all is majestic. But, when a climber was stuck on an overhanging ledge, had lost part of her climbing gear including her two-way radio, and the first in a series of winter storms suddenly invaded the valley, both the climber and her would-be rescuers were stranded. There was nowhere to turn; a helicopter couldn't get close to the climber because the wind and snow were already so turbulent. The climber, a bit too inexperienced, had started somewhat underprepared, without warm enough clothing for a storm, and with food and water for only a few days.

For that climber, a straightforward climbing challenge, beginning from the top of El Capitan, suddenly became a nightmare of considerations: equipment, clothing, food, nightfall, temperature, wind, cramps in one leg, and outjutting of rock just barely long enough to stand on: all in all a technical challenge for which she was not prepared. The majesty of El Capitan became a web of horrors.

For the physician, at the outset of a treatment the field of operations also may look uncomplicated. Part way into the clinical trek, however, the terrain often begins to change. Not that all the excitement turns to horror, but the physician's original clarity becomes murky, handholds familiar from past treatments for similar disorders disappear, and, for the moment at least, the landscape may seem impassible. At the point, ironically, when he or she is least able to do so, the physician, like our climber, may need to reorient and calculate into his or her "mapping" the multiplying factors influencing the treatment. Here, again, we are confronted with the need for strategy in clinical work.

The team perspective comes into this example with the rescue effort. In the case of the climber it took several days to strategize and manage the rescue, because of the storms and the fact that three of the rescue workers were injured during that operation. By the way, it was not easy to recruit all of the rescue workers on a moment's notice, and two had to leave the team mid-course because of other obligations.

The challenge for every physician, as well as team members and the collaborating patient, is, of course, doing the right thing from point to point as they traverse their particular treatment terrain. But, as you can see, facing this task is not likely to be straightforward or easy. Solomon's private decision to let things go while his body deteriorated, or Alan's to "play" for the last several months of his life are cases in point. Neither patient shared their agenda with physicians or even family members since they anticipated unfriendly responses. New medical, personal, and psychological considerations become prominent as treatment moves on, and the MPCP has the job of recognizing and incorporating all of them into the treatment plan and strategy.

Back to strategy, again

What does all this – the specific and frequently convoluted configuration created by the interaction of the physician and patient – have to do with clinical strategy? Of course, everything.

Strategy in primary care and its interface with psychiatry: Solomon

Return again to Solomon. It is true that Solomon believed he had at most a few years left to live when I began to work with him. In fact, that was part of his previously alluded-to "secret": convictions about his health that he kept private since his son and daughter-in-law were convinced that he was being "dramatic" and attempting to play on their sympathies. He was sharp, could see the deterioration in his body, and was acutely aware of the expansion of medical specialists required for him to get adequate care. As far as he was concerned the handwriting was on the wall. That I was so interested in his personal and medical welfare gave him hope. But, Solomon, raised with stoic parents on a Minnesota farm, was absolutely insistent on being "realistic" about his future.

Strategy in Solomon's treatment? What should that have been, and, if he had already signed out, why go to the trouble of being strategic anyway? The answer is that what Solomon felt at a given moment was tentative. His mood at that point was most likely influenced by despair about his wife's leaving the marriage for another man, in part a reaction to his disfigurement caused by scleroderma. Additionally, in contention with Solomon, his son and daughter-in-law insisted he move from his comfortable home in Louisiana to a retirement community located near them in the San Francisco Bay Area. Their claim was that, since he was now alone so much of the time, he would be better off there. Add these facts to what you already know about him. This information (improving our truing) changes things, doesn't it? So, was Solomon giving up because of his progressing medical condition or just feeling defeated and coerced? These are never simple judgments.

My joining Solomon in the what he claimed were "realistic" aspects of his despair would probably have been OK in itself and readily accepted by him. However, I believe people should have repeated opportunities to reconsider positions about their own fate. But what if, like Solomon, the signals they send are somewhat ambiguous? Given a chance to reconsider his position, might Solomon have preferred to fight for his life and dignity rather than yield to the despair that was progressively immobilizing him?

Begin with diagnosis: Solomon was ill. His skeletal system and internal organs were becoming affected. He was crippled with hip problems. In addition to skin, esophagus, and stomach involvement, he was beginning to develop pulmonary fibrosis. At first he was despondent, but over time he became clinically depressed. The primary factors moving him into depression were not entirely clear, however. Candidates included his illness and the attendant disfigurement, the loss of his marriage, being forced to leave his home in Louisiana, and the despotism of his son and daughter-in-law. Mild dementia or even his compromised pulmonary functioning with attendant abnormalities of his blood gases also had to be ruled out. Finally, there were his temperament and his cultural background, all supporting a preference for stoicism and social withdrawal.

Which of these factors would you as the treating physician take up first? How would you make your differential diagnosis, strategize your interventions, and track them? How would you handle the son and daughter-in-law? They regularly disagreed with my opinion that Solomon was not exaggerating his disability, and Solomon believed they were contributing to his lack of motivation through their judgmental attitude. While ostensibly well-meaning, they constantly got in the way of most of our efforts to restore Solomon's sense of self-agency.

The work itself, the strategy

(1) First, I needed to get Solomon on my side. There was more than Solomon's medical and cosmetic decline at issue. Implicated were also the absolute repudiation by his wife, and his son's and daughter-in-law's despotism. These factors clearly contributed to Solomon's withdrawal, moving him to the brink of paranoia about trusting anyone who could meddle with his life. As he sank into despondency and then major depression, Solomon had stopped caring for himself and about his future.

My approach to reintroducing structure and meaning in Solomon's life included the following interventions.

I initially took over many of the essential functions Solomon was neglecting and might otherwise have managed by himself, including the following:

(a) I organized a medical team, communicating with its members regularly. I arranged and at times attended Solomon's medical appointments. I also tracked whether Solomon went to these appointments and followed up assiduously with the involved physicians.

(b) To minimize cancelled meetings I frequently held psychiatric sessions at Solomon's apartment. Solomon had trouble walking and tended to use that as an excuse for avoiding appointments with his physicians, including myself.

(c) I did what I could to discover practical measures to enrich Solomon's, by now, severely impoverished personal life. For example, I bought and assembled a table and organizer for Solomon's computer when it became clear that he was not carrying through on his resolution to maintain his Louisiana connections by learning to use the Internet. The Internet was the main way Solomon's aging friends communicated with one another.

(2) Second, I worked at securing his family's cooperation, talking with Solomon's son weekly, and meeting with his son and daughter-in-law periodically.

(3) Third, I made the decision to be entirely open with Solomon about my opinion of the son's and daughter-in-law's critical attitude. This openness paid off handsomely, creating a "constructive collusion" between Solomon and me. In response, Solomon opened up. He began to confide about his rage toward his, by now, estranged wife. This exercise helped Solomon in his struggle to let go of his failed 40-year marriage. He also began to see me as an ally in his effort to steady himself within the torrent of the family's criticism.

(4) Fourth, and critically important, I established a regular liaison with Solomon's internist who had found it impossible to coordinate this treatment by himself.

(5) Finally, I arranged for psychometric, personality and neuropsychological, assessment. My primary objective was to gain test-based information about Solomon's cognitive status and decisional capacity. If the results supported my impression that his judgment was intact, my plan was to counter his family's allegation that he was incapable of making sound decisions.

Solomon's case became a prototypical medical–psychiatric team effort, with me in two roles: as Solomon's psychiatrist and MPCP. As Solomon's psychiatrist, in addition to providing "reality based" psychotherapy, I used creative measures to demonstrate to him that I understood his position and was on his side in his struggle to free himself from his son and daughter-in-law's tyranny. Having appointments at his apartment and meeting with him for lunch are examples of my attempts to facilitate this kind of interpersonal joining. As MPCP I organized and coordinated his team of medical experts, bringing in each one as needed. In addition, I maintained a close liaison with his son and daughter-in-law, working to help them moderate their demands and criticisms.

Note, the multiplicity of strategic decisions – variety of people and their individual psychologies and possible biases – at work in this case. Each participant contributed a separate point of view about what measures to take in treatment; each potentially introduced a different sensibility.

The outcome as it unfolded

Solomon had two serious falls in his apartment. He could not move well enough with the use of his upper body to right himself, and remained in that helpless state until an attendant came hours later. In both situations he did not call anyone, not his primary care physician, not his son. This was his "who cares" attitude, stoic and characteristic of Solomon at that time. Both incidents occurred toward the beginning of my work with Solomon. They provided a persuasive argument for an even closer liaison among Solomon, myself, and his treatment team, undercutting Solomon's bravado about being self-sufficient.

As I took over his care, Solomon slowly began to open up with me. He started to look forward to our meetings, becoming progressively interested in understanding "our strategy" for managing his son and daughter-in-law and dealing with the emotional impact of his losses. On his own, he began to write down and save his usually concise thoughts and dreams for meetings with me, and we used these as a device for viewing his emotional struggles and tracking his progress in that area. The catastrophic impact of his failed marriage and forced move were the main themes.

Six months later, Solomon began to emphatically stand up to his son and daughter-in-law. He resisted their insistence that he have nursing and hygienic care each day. Defying their orders, he began to bathe only when he wanted to. His dissident behavior was bothersome to his family, but it empowered Solomon.

A few months later, with this experience under his belt, Solomon's interest in self-care began to improve. Solomon, the internist, and I anticipated this shift as we created our strategy. We believed that giving Solomon a greater hand in directing his own life was likely to restore the self-determination he had always prized. At first he made an appointment with a dermatologist by himself. He soon began to call his internist and alert me when there were new medical problems. In turn his mood started to improve. That is, his mood with everyone but his son and daughter-in-law. Stated succinctly, as a response to the strategy he, his internist, and I authored, Solomon became more compliant with treatment, happier in general, and more assertive with his son and daughter-in-law.

The ultimate outcome

As stated earlier, Solomon had been right all along. Indeed, as he had at first discerned, he really did only have a rather short time to live. He was beginning to experience acceleration in organ failure. Most concerning was the progressing involvement of his lungs. Moving forward many months, what ultimately killed him was a septicemia originating in infected skin lesions. Nonetheless, life was better. His Louisiana friends had finally visited, but, according to Solomon's wishes, stayed in California for just two days. For the first time, also, he began to take real pride in his grandchildren.

At this point, you are probably beginning to catch onto the final piece of strategy Solomon and I orchestrated. All team members were informed and all were in agreement. His son and daughter-in-law, however, never fully got on board. Solomon, like the initial Keith, was actually resigned as he contemplated his by now truncated future. He had the relative isolation he asked for; all the medical support he needed to mitigate his pain and suffering was in place, and there were by now a few satisfying relationships in his life, including ours. In response to the sudden deterioration in his health, he said he preferred to die rapidly and not sit by to watch his body continue to fall apart. He had gotten the necessary reprieve, and that was enough for this very proud but private man.

The last challenge during his final weeks was managing his incredulous son and daughter-in-law, who were still having trouble believing Solomon was as sick as the medical members of the team insisted. And, so, Solomon and I dealt with this piece by ourselves. The son and daughter-in-law cooperated to a point but still made Solomon's life a bit uncomfortable through the end. Nonetheless, Solomon listened less and less to them and more to himself.

Solomon seemed relatively tranquil when he was admitted to the intensive care unit (ICU) for the last time. According to him, this was a reasonable, and I believe not surprising, ending for his life.

Strategy in psychiatry: Neal

Recall the following list of "imponderables" from earlier in this chapter. These were offered as additions to the list of "the major personal contributions of physician and patient to the clinical process" from Chapter 6. These, once again, are:
(1) unspoken agendas contributed individually by the physician and patient, including the personal biases, transferences, and countertransferences the patient and physician bring to bear as they work;
(2) the physician's and patient's personal limitations, many idiosyncratic and related to his or her background;

(3) cultural considerations influencing both the physician and patient;
(4) current events in each participant's life;
(5) biological influences on the physician's and patient's state of mind;
(6) the personal and formal theories the physician and patient hold about how change occurs thorough interpersonal influence in treatment.

As we review the strategy SAF used with Neal, note that all of these items are constantly in play.

Neal came from an educated, middle-class background, half Catholic and half Jewish. His parents differed on the value of introspection, his father matter of fact and mother always focused on emotions. Their differences confused him, even at age 22. As you know, Neal could not sit still for over an hour and was always brimming with ideas. When I (SAF) met him he was feeling defeated, having dropped out of college twice, and was defensive about the subject. He hated seeing me at first and I felt similarly about him. And so it went.

Life outside the physician's office is less clear-cut than may be apparent from a brief description of a patient's background, like this one. It is complicated by myriad of real-life influences. That certainly was the case for Neal, for whom the idea of receiving psychiatric treatment made absolutely no sense. Nonetheless, Neal needed help and had no idea what it might do for him. The edict from his parents that he try it drew nothing from him at first but irritation.

So, what to do? What would you have done?

Here are my impressions and the corresponding parts of my initial clinical strategy as it evolved. Note the judgments that were required at each point, and the often subjective nature of the data I used to arrive at these.

(a) I both needed information about Neal's psychology and felt clear about the importance of establishing myself as a serious presence in his life. Yet I had the sense that I couldn't ask too many probing questions without distancing him.
(b) But, I couldn't just stand by. Neal was sinking and I had to do something.
(c) I felt that I had to make myself credible to Neal. Neal respected intelligence, so what I said had to be convincing to him. It seemed important that I be accurate most of the time.

   I couldn't be a "soft-headed psychology type," since he didn't respect that quality in people.
(d) Neal repeatedly challenged me to prove my value to him. If I promised to deliver a message to his parents, such as one about his requiring a car when he returned to school, I did it. If he was worried about headaches and I promised to contact a neurologist and chase down the results of the MRI of his cervical spine, I did it. In my judgment, in order to build and retain Neal's commitment to the treatment, each assignment had to be carried out quickly, with me reporting back to Neal.
(e) I felt that I needed to be flexible about meeting times. As a result, some of our sessions lasted for only 20 minutes, at least at the beginning of our work.

When a session was beginning to drag, we both felt it, and in many cases I decided to bring the meeting to an early close.

(f) Neal seemed strangely tolerant about my talking to his parents, possibly because he despaired of personally making a successful case with them about his typically idiosyncratic aspirations and plans. So, I made the best out of this collaboration, and, as well, used my position to advise his parents to withhold support if Neal tried to move away or terminate treatment prematurely.

Tracking Neal's treatment

Of course, you can't claim you have come up with a successful strategy unless you can prove it. Was Neal progressing? What was the evidence? Was his life any more on track now as compared to the way it was when we began to work together? One criterion psychotherapists justifiably use in evaluating their work is the quality of the patient–therapist relationship. However, while this factor, a strong treatment alliance, figures heavily in a patient's commitment to treatment, without changes in other life sectors it may not generalize and result in basic changes in mood and attitude (Folensbee, 2007).

Here is what I (SAF) found out as I probed. Each category below includes an SO appraisal in parentheses.

(1) Neal was becoming less irritable with his parents and his friends. (Other: improved interest in others.)

(2) He was less intolerant of real-life demands like getting and holding a job. In fact, he was successfully employed in three part-time jobs by a year into treatment. (Self: change in expectations of self.)

(3) After about a year of treatment Neal claimed that he was prepared to re-enter college. He was realistic in acknowledging his lack of enthusiasm for the prospect but also in recognizing that he had no choice if he was going to progress in life. Neal also had committed himself to 10 twice-weekly treatment sessions consisting of cognitive behavioral psychotherapy combined with psychoeducation, and aimed at addressing his ADHD. About midway through this series he dropped his characteristic contempt for psychology and grudgingly acknowledged that the treatment was helpful to him. (Self: Neal was becoming more realistic and usefully introspective; a measure of progress in his "sense of self.")

(4) Neal was beginning to be a bit more sociable. For the first time since I'd met him he admitted that he did not like being by himself all the time. When he initially came for treatment he reported always feeling uncomfortable when with people. He described himself at that point as being "painfully shy." (Self with other: improved sociability.)

(5) Overall, Neal seemed less inclined to blame others for his failures and more willing to discuss them. (This impression, belonging in the "composite" SO category, is best thought of as related to the stability of the patient's self concept and ability to make rational judgments.)

The measures I used to track Neal relied on his reporting and my personal judgment: our collaboration. Throughout our year and a half of work together, I privately tracked him using the SO framework, impressed that the depth and texture of his relationships as well as his self-esteem were evolving. At first, with only collaborative feedback and my clinical and SO appraisals available to monitor Neal, I could not be sure if a shift in his basic attitude was occurring. Providing the required clarification was the last truing measure available to us, psychometric assessment.

The product: the final strategy

The following is a retrospective summary of the clinical strategy at which I arrived and its evolution as Neal progressed. Let's take this subject from bottom up, the initial developments first. Note how clinical judgment determines strategy.

(1) Neal was at first personally inaccessible; he was not in favor of treatment, and for that matter he did not want any intrusion into his private life. So, the first strategic task was to find a way to get Neal to join with me. I needed not just to inform him about what treatment was about but to also to make it credible to him.

(2) Second, Neal was uninterested in the treatment; so, the second task was, like it or not, to make treatment interesting to him. It helped as we worked toward this goal that I progressively found Neal interesting to work with, as well.

(3) Third, I needed to have something technical to offer Neal. In this case that consisted of my knowledge of ADHD, my ability to prescribe psychostimulant medication, my leverage with Neal's parents, my insight into the origins of Neal's chronic pessimism, and my ability to work with Neal to anticipate life developments. Neal was particularly interested in my observations about how his older brother's successes had become a burden for him and how his ADHD constantly thwarted his efforts to be effective in and out of school.

(4) Fourth, I had to play my cards close to the vest; Neal's self-esteem was fragile. As a result, I needed to be careful about showing him how much I knew about his psychology in order not to subvert his tenuous conviction that he understood himself best and had the ultimate control over his life.

(5) While Neal became progressively more involved in treatment and willing to cooperate, he only accepted partial responsibility for initiating changes in his life. Granted, returning to school was his idea, and a monumental one at that. But as a measure of his continued ambivalence about moving on in his life, I had to remind him to call the college academic advisor well in advance of the beginning of the school.

These were the strategic requirements as they emerged with Neal. As in most "real life" cases there was no direct route from the initial assessment to treatment results. Different itineraries become evident with every patient. In each case these evolve with time. It is interesting to compare the personal nature of these individualized roadmaps to the fixed protocols of an EBT or EST.

The outcome

You know already how it went with Neal. He returned to college. This was the small, academically competitive institution he was forced to leave a year and a half earlier. According to him and his parents, and in language uncharacteristic of the early Neal, "things went pretty well." He found a girlfriend during the first year and graduated the following winter. He occasionally initiated contact with me when he needed guidance. It seems reasonable to conclude that the strategy I used – the decision to at first focus on engaging Neal while at the same time collaborating with his parents and then to move into a collaborative role in the treatment – succeeded.

Truing in perspective

Back to the question of how a physician can most successfully find his or her way through the clinical morass that so regularly reveals itself as a case unfolds. We know that truing helps. We have touched particularly on three means of truing in the case descriptions in this chapter. All are practical and can be readily used in office-based practice. These methods are: (1) collaboration with the patient, utilizing the feedback that accrues in that process; (2) physician self-monitoring with devices like repeat history taking and clinical examinations, laboratory tests, and the SO framework; (3) psychometric assessments ranging from easy-to-use and inexpensive self-report and symptom inventories to psychologist-administered tests that are more complex and costly. We are left with the lingering question about how accurate these methods are, singly or in combination, for diagnostic assessment and treatment monitoring. "Incremental validity" provides a partial answer. A multiplicity of truing measures and their repetition as treatment progresses is likely to provide more accurate and useful information than individual measures that are used only once or twice during a treatment.

The MPCP perspective

The previous section deals with psychiatric and systemic medical treatment as a two-person endeavor. Honestly, however, we once again ask, how reasonable is it to think of any complex treatment in this way? What would have happened to Solomon's treatment if his internist had referred him to an immunologist for an independent consultation and the immunologist wrote one of those "Thank you very much for referring Mr. X" notes? The note would finish with recommendations. In Solomon's case these would most likely have been that no specific treatment for his scleroderma was in order at that time but that his diet-based anemia needed attention. The follow-up appointment would be scheduled in six months. The internist could implement that treatment recommendation. It would be straightforward enough. But, given Solomon's passivity, what do you imagine would have happened over that period of time to his general welfare, his poor hygiene and festering skin lesions, and his mourning and troubled relationship with his family as they affected his health?

The point is that this treatment, as most complex treatments, became a team effort by virtue of the multiple physicians and healthcare professionals involved in the work. The team, whether or not constituted formally, consists of both professional and non-professional, collaborating members. Teams, however, need direction. Leaderless teams loose efficiency. Further, not just any leader will do. In Solomon's case that person needed to have the ability to formulate and use group as well as individual psychology as he or she evaluated the team's progress and Solomon's needs. The team in this case included Solomon, his family members as collaborators and participants, his internist, his immunologist, his dermatologist, and other physicians who eventually became integral to the treatment team.

Sound simple? But, wait. The immunologist had at first been irritated with Solomon's reticence, thinking of him as uncooperative. He also did not yet see the point of teamwork in this case. It would simply be another time drain for him. Later, once the immunologist did engage with the team, Solomon's son nonetheless found a "bone to pick with him." That development required the MPCP's and team's time and attention so it would not further obstruct treatment progress.

This case also illustrates why it is preferable and often essential for the coordinator in complex cases like this – cases with significant psychiatric–systemic medical co-morbidity – for the MPCP to be a physician, and, when psychiatric issues are prominent, a psychiatrist. How effective do you think a non-physician case manager would be at understanding the pathophysiology and psychiatric consequences of Solomon's medical and interpersonal situation? Could that person have communicated effectively with the other team members, physicians included? When Solomon's septicemia quickly became an emergency, he had to be admitted to the ICU. Could someone without physician's training have competently negotiated that situation and anticipated its personal impact on Solomon?

So, it seems eminently reasonable to focus on the specific requirements of the MPCP's role. It is the MPCP's job to determine whether the case is being managed and is moving along adequately. From the start, the MPCP needs to be sure each team member makes his or her outcome criteria clear and that these goals are compatible with the objectives set for the case altogether. It helps for the MPCP to identify which truing measures each team member will depend upon, recognizing that this list is likely to evolve over time. And, finally, the MPCP has the job of tracking the product of each team member's effort, as well as that of the team collectively, always with an eye on the ultimate goal: results.

It is not unusual for individual team members to have different criteria for success. Solomon was interested in a rapid, pain-free end for his life. The internist had no choice but to focus on management of Solomon's multiple systemic illnesses. His thinking needed to incorporate current standards of care and he could not have fully cooperated with Solomon's desire to stop fighting for his life. Solomon's son and daughter-in-law were mainly interested in proving that Solomon was exaggerating his disability. Success to them always involved Solomon returning to his original, only minimally disabled self. SAF, as the MPCP, needed to pick and choose among these criteria, strategically deciding which should be adopted to guide the team's efforts and when to bring each one into play.

In the end, Solomon's criterion was selected as the prevailing measure since his lack of flexibility had been tested and no other outcome was agreeable to him. Once that decision was made, SAF needed to work with the other team members to have them accept and follow the revised guidelines. He was successful in this mission with all team members except Solomon's son and daughter-in-law, whose goals remained in partial conflict with the team through the end.

Strategy?

So, as you can see, the MPCP is first and foremost a strategist, technically and interpersonally. The training and skills for this role are manifold. The personality traits required are important as well. The MPCP needs to enjoy solving the complex puzzles that systemic medical and psychiatric problems pose in a multi-person, multi-systems context. He or she needs to have excellent negotiating skills. In addition to currency with primary care medicine and psychiatry, he or she is in effect in part each: an organizational psychologist who can focus on social systems and their impact on individual patients; a psychotherapist who understands behavioral techniques and individual as well as group psychology; a psychopharmacologist; and a medical statistician who knows how to frame and measure clinical progress. It is no wonder, then, that we believe a psychiatrist, with broad interests that include systemic medicine, is the physician of choice for the MPCP role and most particularly for cases involving the kinds of complex patients about which we write.

8

Working consensus: the importance of physician–patient collaboration

It would be gratifying if life, including clinical life, could be broken down into simple cause and effect sequences. We've known a lot of people who believed they could maintain this stance, but virtually none for whom it has worked in the long run. Confounding life, for example, are little irritating intrusions like ambition, taxes, and illness. Complicating the course of an illness are new symptoms, side effects, and discouragement. Family members meddle and complain. Treatment teams are difficult to coordinate as members disagree with one another or drift away.

Over and above his or her own skills in diagnosis and facilitating clinical engagement, is the entire range of experience and sensibilities a physician brings to a treatment. Something similar is true for the patient, who is wise, influential, and, yes, biased in his or her own way. As an analogy to clinical complexity, think of a map of Australia. From above Australia is a single entity, a subcontinent. However, it is also a disparate collection of geographic and ethnic distinctions. Within these divisions there are towns and cities, each of which is in some way different. Then there are the individual families: the structure and peculiarities of each. The complexity, when you care to see it, is nearly infinite.

A multiplicity of clinical issues: Solomon

Back to patients. Evidence-based treatments and empirically supported treatments have a way of making the clinical landscape look uncomplicated. But, how often have you encountered a decision tree that tells the whole clinical story?

First, Solomon. In addition to scleroderma, he suffered from a number of other systemic medical and psychiatric illnesses. Always at hand for his treatment team was the problem of which entity to take on, and when. There were, of course, the multiple complications of scleroderma, including skin lesions that required regular debridement. At the point he came to SAF for treatment, he required TPN feeding for gastrointestinal complications that included dysphagia and immobility of his fibrotic esophagus. Not mentioned in our descriptions of Solomon so far, and complicating the problem of maintaining his nutrition, Solomon had a long-standing eating disorder consisting of compulsive fasting to prevent weight gain.

Reviewing history you already know, Solomon had two hip replacements during the five years prior to referral. These procedures resulted in substantial pain and limitation of movement; so his ability to walk was severely restricted. More recently added problems included pulmonary fibrosis, skin lesions that for the first time were becoming infected, and periods of apparent loss of consciousness responsible for falls from which he could not right himself. Complicating his personal life was the recent loss of his 40-year-long marriage and a forced move from Louisiana to California putting him in closer proximity to his always critical son and daughter-in-law. This move significantly limited his access to a long-standing group of friends and his physicians.

In this chapter we want to emphasize how, in complex cases, physicians, healthcare workers, and the patient and family repeatedly arrive at points of consensus about which issues to deal with and how that work should be done. Relevant in Solomon's case is how Solomon and I (SAF) found our way through the maze of his medical and personal problems, especially as Solomon's resistance to treatment grew.

Diagnostic ambiguity: Alison

Alison was an unhappily married mother of three who worked as a radiologist. In her early life she had allegedly been abused by her parents and molested sexually by her grandfather. Alison came to SAF hoping to deal with the psychological consequences of these experiences. Because of her "discomfort being starred at," she insisted that treatment sessions be conducted from a location in his office where SAF could not directly see her. Their consensus about the nature and even validity of Alison's difficulties faltered as SAF misinterpreted her unusual request as coquettish.

Begin with the question of Alison's diagnosis. To start with there were several reasonable possibilities. From the DSM-IV-TR they were:

(1) based on her history:

Axis I – Posttraumatic Stress Disorder (309.81), and Dissociative Disorder, Depersonalization type (300.6).

And

(2) based on her presentation:

Axis II – Dependent Personality Disorder (301.6), and Histrionic Personality Disorder (301.5).

However, while these diagnostic categories were consistent with aspects of Alison's presentation, each accounted for only part of her clinical picture. None described Alison fully.

One of SAF's challenges, then, became selecting between diagnostic possibilities, predicting which categories would provide an accurate focus for treatment, and identifying which aspects of her presentation did not fit these or any other standard categories. A diagnostic situation that at first seemed straightforward progressively became foggy.

Truing as it contributes to consensus

So far in this book we have followed the physician as she or he endeavored to negotiate the assessment and treatment process. This activity, involving a series of truing measures, was first outlined in Chapter 2. That odyssey usually begins with referral information. Next, the physician takes a history and conducts a clinical examination. Ideally, more history is gathered over time as it becomes relevant. Then there are formal assessments including physician self-monitoring involving his or her subjective assessment of the patient's status through a device like the SO analysis, symptom checklists, psychometric assessments, diagnostic imaging, and laboratory studies. Some of the original assessments may be repeated later to monitor progress. Added throughout treatment are consultations with other physicians and allied healthcare professionals. Over time, new diagnostic and treatment strategies are evolved to reorient the work as it loses direction or becomes inefficient.

In this chapter we bring back a truing device discussed briefly in Chapter 6: the patient's moment by moment personal judgment about the treatment and the feedback loops he or she establishes with the treating physician. At the MPCP level this activity is expanded to include collaboration with multiple people including team members, the patient, and frequently the patient's family. This interactive activity, when it succeeds, is essential to the development and maintenance of physician–patient consensus.

The consequences of not collaborating with a patient

How much of a contribution to keeping treatment on target can the patient really make? To evaluate this issue, we move to two patients, Nathan, who is new to you, and Keith, whom you met in Chapter 2.

Nathan

Nathan, a 78-year-old, retired concert pianist, came to his internist complaining of inexplicable weakness and some loss of coordination in his lower extremities, as well as alternating constipation and diarrhea. His wife had died 10 years earlier, leaving his personal care to his overbearing daughter. He was tentatively diagnosed at that time with Parkinson's disease and treated with carbidopa/levodopa

(Sinemet). However, his physical examination findings were atypical for Parkinson's disease, and his physicians were confounded by the distribution of his weakness. Uncertainty about the relationship between his bowel symptoms and Parkinson's disease also needed clarification. Digestive problems are common in Parkinson's disease, and the dopaminergic agents commonly used to treat it such as carbidopa/levodopa can themselves cause gastrointestinal dysfunction.[1]

Additionally, and on a different track, was Nathan's emphatic opinion that his weakness and gastrointestinal symptoms were significantly caused by anxiety; in his view based on fear of becoming disabled as his Parkinson's disease progressed. Several years after the initial diagnosis was made and when the results were mostly in, it became clear that Nathan knew what he was talking about. Indeed he had Parkinson's disease, but it had progressed slowly. Anxiety and then depression, affecting his will to live, undoubtedly also played a major role in Nathan's symptoms. Unfortunately, however, in the beginning of his treatment neither the anxiety nor depression was sufficiently addressed, those managing his case apparently not taking his opinion that psychiatric issues played a significant role in his disease very seriously.

Nathan's situation, however, was additionally complicated. As time went on it became clear that, while implicated, neither explanation – not Parkinson's disease nor psychiatric issues – adequately accounted for all of Nathan's symptoms. Throughout treatment, his bowel problems and weakness conspicuously progressed. Neither the manifestations nor extent of either, however, were ever fully explained or contained.

Returning to Keith

From the point of view of medical management, Keith's experience was quite a bit more troubling than Nathan's. Keith was blindsided by his over-zealous internist, Dr. R. As described in Chapter 6, Keith suffered from progressing bone marrow failure, his polycythemia vera eventually converting to leukemia. With the prognosis dire and his cooperation secured, I (SAF) accepted Keith's invitation to help him prepare for his impending death. I was surprised and gratified when he asked to meet with me weekly to help him understand the likely course of his medical condition and prepare him for what he concluded were going to be his final months.

---

[1] Constipation is the most common bowel problem associated with Parkinson's. When related to Parkinson's, constipation has several causes.
  (a) The muscles of the bowel wall can be affected due to problems with mobility and rigidity.
  (b) Lack of movement and exercise means that the bowel is not stimulated to function normally.
  (c) As some people with Parkinson's disease have problems with swallowing, they may be unable to eat a diet with enough fiber.
  (d) Actually emptying the bowel can be a problem: it might be difficult to brace the abdominal muscles to assist bowel emptying, and the anal sphincter may not relax at the right time to allow the stool to be passed easily.

Ironically, as you may remember, the one who could not accept Keith's prognosis and his wish for ongoing dignity was Dr. R., who insisted on painful and heroic measures to keep him alive. These treatments indeed slowed Keith's demise, but soon, perhaps as a result of his rapidly progressing medical condition, Keith began to slip into dementia. Keith's wife and I begged the internist to relent and to let Keith die peacefully. However, in response to these requests the internist became more entrenched in his position and less communicative. Soon Keith became cognitively impaired and thus decisionally incapacitated, losing control and dignity during his dying. His decline and eventual death were hideous.

These two examples, Nathan and Keith, illustrate how not incorporating the patient's input can interfere with proper treatment. Physicians and other health-care professionals are used to depending on their own clinical judgment and test data for direction (Verghese, 2002; Groopman, 2007). Our position, however, is that prominently including the patient's input in this process is a good idea. The joining of minds between the physician and patient – the consensus they arrive at – almost always augments clinical work.

How consensus works: the nuts and bolts

A.   Rapport in treatment

It should be helpful for us to look a bit more closely at the treatment alliance as an essential component in the development of consensus about treatment issues.

Alison: the microscopic picture

This topic, interpersonal contributions to the physician–patient rapport as the prelude for consensus about clinical care, is one of the most elusive with which we will grapple (Elkin et al., 1989; Olges et al., 1995; Krupnick et al., 1996; Barber et al., 2000; Frankel, S., 2000, 2007; Roth & Fonagy, 2005; Hilsenroth, 2007; Pellerin et al., 2011). After all, how do you talk about what, for the most part, you can't see and confirm?

Alison, who was introduced at the beginning of the chapter, would say that she was always going for the feel of things, and I (SAF) know that on a personal level it is similar for me. When I go into the consulting room everything changes. I greet the patient. My eyes widen. I hunch forward feeling for the electromagnetic-like field the patient emits, different each time. With Alison I generally monitored whether she was withdrawn or relaxed, following her mood as it shifted. We might start by talking about her husband, as if those words carried the power between us. Alison would listen for the tension, worry, or softness in my voice and immediately register how present or preoccupied I was. That intensity was essential as together we searched for a shared basis for relating. Much of this activity happened without words. In case this description doesn't sound like it applies to general practice medicine, good physicians notice and respond in these ways all the time, just not usually so deliberately.

Solomon: the macroscopic view

Solomon, you probably recall, originally came from a rural town in Minnesota. In keeping with his cultural background, he tightly regulated his words and emotions. I (SAF) wondered after each visit whether he would return for the next scheduled appointment. Because he was so self-determined and angry at people like his son and daughter-in-law who "wanted to run" his life, Solomon had no intention of fully cooperating with any of his physicians. I was no exception.

Rapport was first evident when, to Solomon's surprise, I took the risk of telling him I agreed that his son and daughter-in-law were being unreasonable by insisting on monitoring his moves. Not only did I openly concur with Solomon about this topic, but I made it clear that I could understand both his decision to restrict his life to basic activities and desire for social isolation. After all, with Solomon's wife's abandonment in the background and the fact that her leaving him was at least partially based on his deteriorating appearance, his waning interest in embracing life made logical sense to me. Solomon needed to be convinced that he and I were allied around these issues before we could take the next step of talking about his needs and future.

Slowly, glacially, Solomon's mood began to improve over time. Our bond and the possibility of our developing a *working consensus* about our goals grew, as did his desire to cooperate with his other physicians. However, there were conditions he implicitly established for our work to be ongoing. I needed to be absolutely reliable about our visits, I had to remember to call him at least once between visits, I had to say "yes" when he invited me to lunch at his retirement facility, and, above all, I needed to be absolutely committed to Solomon's requirement for agency in his relationship with his son and daughter-in-law.

There were also complications as our work gained momentum. As I successfully supported Solomon's prerogative to make his own decisions, the intensity of his son's and daughter-in-law's protests rose. This development became the acid test of Solomon's commitment to treatment and continuation of the progress he had been making. It accentuated the importance to our work of the rapport and consensus we had developed to that point.

B.   Another level of consensus: cooperation between team members

Recall Alan, who at first couldn't "give a plug nickel" for psychiatry. As far as he was concerned, that kind of "hooey" was best relegated to jokes about "shrinks." And yet, as he got to know me (SAF), as his wife began to rail at me as well as at him when things went wrong, and as his breathing began to fail, he started to look forward to our meetings. He brought in "peace offerings": a picture of his children, an old newspaper clipping from his childhood.

Then, out of the blue, I got a call. It was Alan's hematologist. He was encouraged. Alan had finally agreed to consider a bone marrow transplant. Where to go from here? He reiterated the plan that had previously been suspended. He wanted to know if I could help. I explained that the future of the treatment, whether Alan indeed did get the transplant, depended on how well the members of the treatment team could work together. Also, I added, they all needed to embrace Alan's involvement and treat him as a fully collaborating team member.

During that call, the hematologist seemed to understand the specific requirements for Alan's sustained cooperation. We left the talk feeling hopeful. The hematologist said he recognized how Alan's self-indulgent tendencies could get in the way of our treatment success. We talked about our previous lack of consensus and the need to develop a unified plan if we were to succeed this time. However, tragically, the hematologist, who was based at a large university hospital, got too busy to reliably follow-up. Alan needed more than a few appointment cards and calls from medical secretaries to remain engaged. We all, Alan's internist, the hematologist, representatives from the transplant service, and myself had agreed that consistent teamwork would be necessary for the plan to be successfully implemented. We had talked about conference calls and monthly meetings with all team members – great ideas – but, they never happened. In the end the only engaged collaborators were Alan and myself, and Alan, given his impressive capacity to lose himself in frivolity, never received his bone marrow transplant.

C. Further deconstructing the treatment alliance: the physician's distortions

Switch for a moment to Marty, a 40-year-old, retired businessman, who became infuriated with me (SAF) when I charged him for a missed psychiatric session he failed to cancel. Marty was argumentative by nature but was especially adamant in this situation when he insisted that I absolutely "needed to listen" to him. I resisted, convinced that Marty was simply being contentious and possibly trying to take advantage of me; irritated at his accusing tone. Buried in my mind was the fact that I was planning to increase Marty's fee. Inflation-indexed fee increases were a part of my financial arrangement with Marty.

How did I know when to take Marty's argument seriously or to acknowledge Alison's complaint that my resisting her request to sit in a place in my office where I could not see her seemed "mean-spirited" to her? In each case, I eventually made a significant internal shift that allowed me to more clearly hear the patient's point of view. In both situations, the change in my awareness moved me from skepticism to belief, from conditional involvement to commitment. However, on the face of it, the timing and reasons for my shifts seem inexplicable: a mystery that only reference to the most microscopic details of the interaction could clarify.

Similar forces operate all the time in systemic medicine, especially in the treatment of chronic illness where interpersonal frustration is typically magnified. Heartfelt patient compliance with a confusing, painful, and/or costly medical regimen requires more than just initial goodwill on the part of the physician and patient. Sticking with a treatment over years can bring out the best or worst in either.

The details of my interaction with Marty and Alison are what we are driving at when we refer to "deconstructing the treatment alliance." Putting a magnifying glass to my interaction with Alan and Solomon would yield the same kind of interpersonal data. In those cases it was compliance with medical treatment that was at stake. The shifts I am describing for Alison and Marty were not anticipated and, certainly, at the time they occurred were not fully explicable. In each case, the patient's requirements went against my grain, and my own reaction became problematic for the treatment.

Primary care physicians who mainly treat systemic illness may find the described clinical stance impractical: too fraught with detail, the time frame too extended. But, when do you not encounter this kind of complex interpersonal situation in your office or clinic? At first, your patient sees you as a "savior." But then the glow begins to fade. Complaints, then accusations, begin to replace admiration (Gawande, 2003). Your own reactions to the patient begin to interfere with rapport and treatment efficacy. How best to play out this situation, since what you need is cooperation and results: consensus between yourself and the patient? The answer is contained in the above examples, where deconstruction of the clinical situation provides an understanding of exactly what interpersonal issues you are working with. Our claim is that it doesn't matter whether the situation is in primary care or psychiatry; the same principles apply.

A mixed systemic medical–psychiatric case: Natalie

Judging from close up, it seems clear that much of what enables a physician and patient to accurately find their way in a treatment is often neither fully understood nor verbalized. The ways I came to believe and understand Marty's and Alison's claims that I had gotten it wrong, and Solomon's skepticism about the value of accepting direction from me, provide a set of parallels as we embark on my experience of establishing consensus with Natalie.

"Believing" was the single most important theme in my (SAF's) work with Natalie. My difficulty fully trusting the two explanations she offered for her systemic medical and psychiatric symptoms was the limiting factor in our work. The first explanation was about her medical conditions: eczema, serious in childhood; Sjögren's syndrome as an adult.[2] She presented medical data to

---

[2] Sjögren's syndrome is an autoimmune disorder in which immune cells attack and destroy the glands that produce tears and saliva. Sjögren's syndrome is also associated with rheumatic disorders such as rheumatoid arthritis. The hallmark symptoms of the disorder are dry mouth and dry eyes. In addition, Sjögren's syndrome may cause skin, nose, and vaginal dryness, and may affect other organs of the body including the kidneys, blood vessels, lungs, liver, pancreas, and brain.

Sjögren's syndrome affects one to four million people in the United States. Most people are more than 40 years old at the time of diagnosis. Women are nine times more likely to have Sjögren's syndrome than men.

support these diagnoses. Nonetheless, I couldn't help thinking that this woman, rife with physical complaints, was at least a bit of a somatizer.

It was the second explanation, however, that actually threw me. Natalie had been plagued by depression throughout most of her life. She tied her depression to the conviction that she had been repeatedly molested in childhood. It was this certainty that particularly troubled her. This allegation both dogged and ultimately provided the depth for our treatment alliance. The emphasis here, and in the rest of this chapter about consensus in clinical work, is on the word "alliance," not "relationship." Physicians and patients always develop a relationship. They don't always form a goal-directed alliance, however.

My work with Natalie allows us to view the interpersonal details of how treatment alliances are developed and maintained. The principles that emerge, however, can and should be extrapolated to clinically and operationally complex clinical situations; those with multiple participants. Successful work in these cases requires the sustained effort of all concerned to arrive at successive points of consensus about treatment issues.

In the beginning, Natalie and I easily formed the words that articulated our treatment goals, and we seemed to agree about how we would achieve these. I thought I understood Natalie and believed that our clinical challenge would be relatively straightforward. I was to help her understand and to treat her depression, as well as participate in the management of the medical and psychological manifestations of her Sjögren's syndrome. Also, as with Alan and Solomon, I would organize and coordinate her treatment team. For my part, as her psychiatrist, the techniques I used would include psychotropic medication and methodical exploration of her symptoms and background, especially as these related to previous trauma. Natalie was sophisticated about medical and psychological matters, and the issues seemed plain enough.

The second child in a sibship of three, 52 years of age at the time of presentation, Natalie had endured persistently depressed moods and experienced severe, disfiguring eczema attacks since late adolescence. Sjögren's syndrome was diagnosed in her early forties. As an adult she felt fated to suffer alone, believing that if people really knew her litany of complaints they would flee. Her parents had

---

There is no known cure for Sjögren's syndrome, nor is there a specific treatment to restore gland secretion. Treatment is generally symptomatic and supportive. Moisture replacement therapies may ease the symptoms of dryness. Non-steroidal anti-inflammatory drugs may be used to treat musculoskeletal symptoms. For individuals with severe complications, corticosteroids or immunosuppressive drugs may be prescribed.

Sjögren's syndrome can damage vital organs of the body, with symptoms that may remain stable, worsen, or go into remission. Some people may experience only the mild symptoms of dry eyes and mouth; while others go through cycles of good health followed by severe disease. Many patients are able to treat problems symptomatically. Others are forced to cope with blurred vision, constant eye discomfort, recurrent mouth infections, swollen parotid glands, hoarseness, and difficulty in swallowing and eating. Debilitating fatigue and joint pain can seriously impair quality of life. (Excerpted from *Harrison's Principles of Internal Medicine*, Fauci *et al.*, 2008.)

belonged to a fundamentalist religious group whose uncompromising principles included disciplining children through beatings. Natalie believed that this history added to the impact of the alleged molestations. Despite this background, she had done well for herself, becoming a hospital administrator, a respected member of the local medical community, and the mother of three purportedly successful girls.

The issue of sexual molestation emerged soon after we started treatment. Natalie began to focus on the tormenting suspicion that she had been repeatedly molested as a child. No clear memories of molestation experiences, just a nagging hunch at first about her father, and then one of her uncles insisting on having oral sex with her when she was about 10. On hearing this story, all I could do was listen, take more history, and wrestle with my nagging skepticism. At that time concern about "false memories," involving patients' manufactured recollections of childhood molestations, was prominent. Most mental health professionals, including psychiatrists, were on alert, especially vigilant about the need to substantiate patients' stories about events such as these.

But Natalie started to produce data: episodes where she had difficulty breathing, the sense of something heavy pressing on her chest at night, and unexplained bouts of nausea. These symptoms were on the borderline between physical and psychological.[3] Since they were vague they were not always easy to separate from the various non-specific symptoms that characterize Sjögren's syndrome. The breathing difficulty made her rheumatologist wonder about incipient lung involvement. The gastrointestinal symptoms were tentatively attributed to the corticosteroids she was prescribed for her Sjögren's syndrome-related arthritis.

As we worked, however, the impression that part of Natalie's medical picture could be related to the resurgence of traumatic memories gained coherence. The nausea and breathing difficulties increased, but also nightmarish impressions that something large was being crammed down her throat. The dreams she reported began to seem like memories. In several of these dreams, she and her daughters were raped. However, there was nothing incontrovertible, nothing clearly factual, about her account.

Complicating an already confounded picture, there was a probable family crisis that could be set off if Natalie held firm to her allegation of childhood sexual abuse. If we seized on the sensations and dreams as "evidence" that she had been sexually molested, if Natalie believed her evolving story, she felt clear that she would be compelled to confront her father, mother, and uncle. Further, according to Natalie, maintaining any sense of personal integrity would require her to cut her ties with the implicated family members.

---

[3] There is a potential link between stress and atopic dermatitis, and by extension eczema (Hashizume *et al.*, 2005). It is more equivocal whether stress can lead to an exacerbation of Sjögren's syndrome. However, although the reason why stress influences skin conditions is not fully understood, studies linking these conditions to depressed immune function suggest a method through which stress and these medical conditions may be connected.

For me as her psychiatrist, a major issue in this emerging drama was the potential it held for moving me to violate diagnostic and treatment rigor. After all, the "data" Natalie brought forth were entirely subjective. None were confirmed as fact. These considerations, together with my training and experience in child psychiatry, advised caution about accepting patients' claims about previously dissociated childhood traumatic experiences, especially when the claims involved blame.

However, Natalie's protests grew. Depression, eczema, and symptoms of Sjögren's syndrome all escalated, as did the frequency of her impressions of childhood molestations, now elevated to the status of "memories." Certainly, in addition to her systemic medical symptoms, her presentation and complaints were compatible with Posttraumatic Stress Disorder (PTSD) (DSM-IV-TR 309.81), with recollections of alleged childhood sexual abuse intruding regularly both into her waking life and dreams. Confusing for me, however, was that Natalie had a stable interpersonal life and marriage, in addition to impressive professional accomplishments. Dysfunction in these areas is frequently associated with the psychological effects of significant early trauma.

Searching for clarification, I contacted a consultant who specialized in PTSD associated with childhood sexual molestation, and described the case to her. After listening to the details, she said that if I wanted the treatment to succeed my only option was to be *open* to accepting Natalie's claim about molestations. If I didn't take Natalie seriously, our treatment was likely to fail. Natalie would see herself as harboring an awful secret and experience me as afraid to join her in dealing with it. If I accepted her story, and we didn't find clear evidence of molestation, we could work further in psychotherapy and deal with any evidence of childhood sexual abuse if it turned up. According to the consultant, this kind of abuse is so alarming that everyone from the perpetrator to the child victim, parents, and society conspire in perpetuating disbelief (van der Kolk, 1988, 2002; Herman, 1992). The consultant also recommended that Natalie have a full psychological assessment to see if it produced evidence of the trauma Natalie believed had occurred. Earlier, Natalie had refused psychological testing when I suggested it, alleging that my recommendation reflected my distrust of her claims about having been molested.

As I write these words, I feel a bit dismayed about the persistence of my initial disbelief, because it slowed our work and, at the time, discouraged Natalie. In my defense, however, in order for Natalie and me to work effectively I believe she needed me to be forthcoming about my uncertainty. I hold that it was my conversion to believing Natalie's story of childhood trauma – its stark contrast with my initial skepticism – that proved to be the most potent factor in instigating the levels of consensus Natalie and I ultimately reached.

The consultant had been right in encouraging me to be open to considering Natalie's story. The psychological assessment, especially the trauma indices on the MMPI and findings from the Rorschach test, produced abundant evidence of early trauma associated with sexual molestation. These findings served to consolidate our shared view about Natalie's diagnosis and treatment requirements. Our evolving conviction, and indeed consensus, about the molestations was, in fact, experienced as "life-sustaining" by Natalie. According to her wishes, my job ultimately became to "preserve the integrity" of her recollections of her troubled past and continue to "bear witness" to her trauma and its psychological consequences (Peskin, 2012).

Critically important in Natalie's treatment was the conviction that the other was fully committed to our project: all steps in the direction of reinforcing our consensus about Natalie's recollections and deepening our rapport. Regarding my role as MPCP, there was also strong evidence of a relationship between our treatment alliance and Natalie's ability to stick with her systemic medical treatment regimen. As our work progressed, her other physicians commented about how much more consistent Natalie had become with her treatments.

Non-verbal contributions to consensus

For Natalie and me spoken language created a frame to contain and direct our experience. It helped us move from point to point in our formal exploration of Natalie's history of alleged sexual trauma, as well as the personal consequences of her illnesses. But, much of our experience in growing to believe one another and remain committed to our treatment was conveyed non-verbally. Points of both verbal and non-verbal agreement, disrupted by episodes of disaffection, progressively grew into shared, tightly held, convictions about the validity of her claims and value of our work.

Research on interpersonal communication in early childhood and its counterpart in adult life (La Barre, 2001; Beebe & Lachmann, 2002) suggests that people are frequently remarkably accurate in their intuitive understanding of one another. They are often good at bringing themselves into alignment (Frankel, S., 2000). The opposite may be true as well, however, with neither member of the treatment dyad able to accurately cue the other either verbally or non-verbally.

That is what happened between Marty and me when I (SAF) did not want to face my irritation at him and privately blamed him for disrupting our work. His anger and defensiveness made shared understanding temporarily impossible. I did not understand Marty's view and at that point in our work was not particularly motivated to understand it. In these kinds of circumstances arriving at clinical consensus actually is a daunting process.

Returning to Natalie, did she and I actually reach consensus? This is a more complicated question than may be apparent. Reflexively, my inclination would be to say that of course we did. We got along. We discussed and agreed about our manifest goals for treatment: the resolution of her depression, containment of eczema attacks, and attention to the physical and emotional manifestations of her Sjögren's syndrome.

But what, then, about our differences? For a long time they were focused around our starkly opposing opinions about the sexual molestation. Others involved our different levels of concern about censure within the professional community, as well as by Natalie's family.

Where, then, is the consensus here?

Judging from our agreement about manifest treatment goals and our commitment to achieving these, Natalie and I were in consensus. Looking at the matter from the point of view of our initially different opinions about the certainty of the alleged molestations and whether trauma might explain some or even most of her physical symptoms, however, we were often not in consensus. Both positions – agreement and disagreement – were often simultaneously in evidence as we worked together.

Working consensus

This clinical example is instructive as we think about how to usefully define "consensus" in clinical work. If it is to be of value in providing orientation as we work, our version of "consensus" needs to be practical (Rorty, 1991; Strenger, 1991; Renik, 1993). It should be useful and clear, not vague and general. It should incorporate the results of a collaborative truing process carried out between the participants in treatment.

To suit these purposes, then, we propose a new term, "working consensus," to describe the ever-changing meeting of minds that occurs in clinical work. We believe the notion of "working consensus" is more useful for this purpose than the non-qualified term, "consensus." "Working consensus" captures the compromise nature of the dialectal clinical process, making that definition especially applicable to the complex interpersonal joining that is repeatedly required for working productively in most treatments, especially those distinguished by their complexity. There were always significant disagreements between Natalie and me, but in spite of these we were always able to find our way, repeatedly arriving at improved versions of our "working consensus."

We are not, therefore, using the term "working consensus" as synonymous with "agreement." Instead, the kind of consensus to which we are referring reflects a truing effort that has the purpose of keeping a treatment focused and productive, regardless of coexisting interpersonal mismatches. "Working consensus," when interpersonal joining is conceptualized in this way, then, usually involves multiple points of view that are simultaneously in play in treatment; some shared and some at odds.

Summing it up

"Consensus" always involves verbal and non-verbal components. "Working consensus" incorporates levels of agreement and disagreement that are managed by the treatment participants in such a way that a treatment can be maintained and remain productive. What counts in "working consensus" is that the main participants are repeatedly able to move toward the treatment goals. The added charge at the MPCP level involves maintaining consensus among team members, patient, and family, about treatment goals and whether they are being met or revisions are needed.

Conventional truing measures are used by team members operating at Level 1 for providing direct treatment to the patient. Truing at the treatment team level, Level 2, is different. (See Chapter 1 for elaboration of our use of the designations "Level 1" and "Level 2.") It includes at least two components, each contributing to the attainment of a consensus that establishes direction for the treatment team. The first involves the MPCP in the role of monitoring treatment results and providing feedback to the team members about movement toward treatment goals. The second consists of the MPCP regularly soliciting feedback from all members of the team, including the patient and at times the family, and using this information to move the treatment forward.

In Chapter 9 we will return for another, more detailed, look at the truing process.

9

Linking truing measures: technical and interpersonal precision in work with complex cases

"Truing" refers to how a physician finds his or her way clinically, moving toward the "truth" about a patient's condition and identifying the best ways to treat. Clinical judgment with its roots in clinical experience (EBCJ) helps to provide direction for that work. However, the validity of these judgments is only established through the monitoring of treatment progress and outcome. Setting outcome measures and following progress are, of course, two truing devices. We began to discuss the concept of truing and its clinical applications in Chapters 1, 2 and 8. In this chapter we take it up in more detail.

Other truing devices in clinical work include: interviews and physical examinations; self-assessment procedures such as serial SO analyses; laboratory tests and diagnostic imaging; psychometric testing; consultations from other health professionals; and interviews with informants such as the patient's spouse, parents, or even, at times, employers. Literature reviews and discussions with colleagues provide additional direction. Granted, none of these truing devices, including laboratory reports, are perfectly objective, but the more sources of information a physician has for understanding and following a case, the greater the chance of finding a reliable direction.

Divergence in findings, of course, may be useful as well. For example, when the physical examination or clinical interview conflict with test findings and a conventional explanation is not at hand, a new explanation is called for. That was the case with Michael, the 16-year-old, diabetic patient who is described below. On interview, Michael's claim was that the diabetes neither bothered nor affected him. His blood tests argued otherwise, however. The diagnostic and clinical challenge seemed straightforward enough; that is, if you failed to take into consideration Michael's "blackouts" during the past several months. Hyperglycemia, even progressing to the point of ketoacidosis, did not fully explain these episodes.

Another source of truing, emphasized in Chapter 8, is physician–patient collaboration. Deliberate attention to creating this exchange with the patient contributes invaluable, albeit anecdotal, feedback about whether the patient is benefitting from treatment. This method of truing also provides assurance that the physician and patient are working according to the patient's, not just the physician's, wishes. Trial periods of treatment strategy round off the list. The physician and patient use these to set and revise goals as treatment progresses.

Formal truing measures versus clinical judgments developed through "the conjunctive sequence"

What is the relationship among formal interviews, test-based data, and the experience-informed judgments (EBCJs) physicians use to guide themselves? In *Making Psychotherapy Work: Collaborating Effectively with Your Patient* (2007), SAF breaks this dimension of treatment into a series of interpersonal activities that builds toward physician–patient alliance. He calls this progression the *conjunctive sequence* (Frankel, S., 2007). The term "conjunction," as used here, refers to points in treatment where the physician and patient have become like-minded about objectives and techniques. While physician–patient compatibility fuels the *conjunctive sequence*, the competence of both parties to grapple with the technical issues that complicate their effort plays a large part in determining how well they work together.

> The *conjunctive sequence* (Frankel, S., 2007) consists at minimum of events designated: (1) "incipient conjunction" (a state of optimism, associated with early treatment, that is shared by physician and patient about the value of their working together), (2) "discovery that the other is different from the person you expected him or her to be" (an occurrence typical for almost any ongoing professional relationship), (3) "controlled disorientation" (a technique available to physician or patient for detecting the other's unspoken agendas), (4) "collaborative feedback between physician and patient" (a largely non-verbal, information-sharing process always at work in treatment), (5) "disruptions and repairs in the working relationship" (with emphasis on their value for initiating new perspectives for the treatment), and (6) "the leap of inference" (a judicious and well-timed statement or action that is instrumental in bringing the clinical work forward).

Clinical illustration: Michael

Here we turn again to Michael, the 16-year-old patient introduced above with diabetes mellitus, unexplained "blackouts," and, in addition, a conduct disorder involving risk-taking. I (SAF) was called in following a serious episode where Mike's blood glucose rose to 325 mg/dL because he defiantly went on a drinking binge with friends and engaged in an orgy of eating junk food.

The first order of business in this situation was obviously to bring Michael's diabetes under control. The second was to find out why he allowed this situation to develop in the first place and create a relationship with Michael that would promote his cooperation with his medical treatment. As you can probably guess, Michael was only half interested in understanding his diabetes. He was "sick and tired of being weird," and didn't exactly buy into his physicians' caution that the disease was progressive and life-long. He didn't want to hear the facts.

It went like this: "Mike, for God's sake listen to me, what's wrong with you, man? Keep this up and you're dust. Don't you get it?"

Unfortunately, my approach was a sure formula for creating a glazed look on Michael's face. And why? Even a 16-year-old is likely to be smarter and wiser than that.

Where could I go from here? I turned to an SO analysis to see what new perspective about Mike's psychology I could come up with. That helped. I already knew that the most important "self" and "other" components for Mike were his intense desire to be "normal" and his preoccupation with social success. His illness interfered with his wish for a "real" 16-year-old life consisting of friends, sports, sex, and free access to drugs and alcohol. So, why should he listen to me or his parents? Acknowledgment of his "defect," the reality of his diabetes, threatened to throw Mike into an abyss of confusion and discouragement. In this case I came onto the scene as the enemy: a physician who brought only unwelcome news.

Here's how the conjunctive sequence went with Michael.

(1) For the most part, Mike and I had bypassed the incipient, "honeymoon" phase that usually provides a smooth entry into most physician–patient relationships. (Incipient Conjunction.)

(2) Shortly after we started, Mike's radar for adult oppression signaled to him that I might not be the helpful, encouraging soul he had assumed that I was. Mike's self-appointed job quickly became to resist rather than listen to me and my advice. (Discovery that the Other is Different from who you Expected or Wanted that Person to be.)

(3) I then needed to search for new ways to understand Mike, novel perspectives that would help me work more effectively with him. At this point the SO analysis often benefits from the deliberate use of "controlled disorientation," a technique for replacing an older view of the patient with a current and more clinically useful one. (Controlled Disorientation.)

(4) The next step was for me to negotiate a reconciliation with Mike, making clear that I meant no harm and might even be able to help make his life better. (Collaborative Feedback between Physician and Patient.)

(5) Of course, that wasn't the end of our troubles. Of necessity, the treatment alliance repeatedly grew and deteriorated. The hope always was that Michael might emerge more comprehending of our work and his medical needs as he weathered these disruptions and their repairs. (Disruption and Repair of the Treatment Alliance.)

(6) All during this time I was also looking for openings to make the kind of statements or deliberate shifts in my delivery that would qualify as "leaps of inference." Preparing for these opportunities with Michael required my

listening to his endless descriptions of sexual escapades with a friend's girl-friend, how "cool they were," or how he and his friends eluded the police after stealing a bottle of wine from a convenience store. After these exchanges, Michael, reassured about my good will, permitted me to make statements about the importance of regulating his blood glucose. At these moments he could entertain the idea that "controlling blood sugar would mean staying out of the hospital and living longer." (Leap of Inference.)

As you can see from this example, the *conjunctive sequence* is essentially a microscopic breakdown of the steps required to effect a meaningful interpersonal connection in the clinical setting. Distinguishing this relationship is that the interacting partners progressively develop a shared view about the value as well as direction and goals of their clinical interaction.

Natalie

For a second illustration using the conjunctive sequence, we return to Natalie. As time passed, my (SAF's) truing efforts were paying off. Assisted by the results of psychometric testing and the consultant's opinion about the ongoing conse-quences of childhood sexual molestations, I was progressively finding Natalie's story credible. It was as if I first had to be encouraged and then force myself to embrace (in effect using "controlled disorientation") Natalie's perspective. Early in our work Natalie recognized that I was dissembling in claiming I wholeheartedly believed her about the molestations and even the validity of her medical symptoms (most likely an instance where the patient's effort to discern my attitude was assisted by her own version of "controlled disorien-tation"). In fact, later, even with several informative truing measures operative, I still was slow to fully embrace Natalie's claims.

It was only with Natalie's verbal and non-verbal confrontations about my lack of authenticity that I was able to regain my bearings (the result of productive "collaborative feedback between physician and patient," preceded by a confron-tation by her). As described in Chapter 8, it was at this point that Natalie accepted my recommendation for psychological personality assessment (an example of "leap of inference" involving my seizing the moment to again raise the issue of assessment). As time went on, agreements and disruptions in the treatment accrued, growing into shared convictions about treatment issues and their man-agement (the product of "disruptions and repairs" in the clinical process).

The personal and interpersonal operations of the *conjunctive sequence* are by nature infused with subjectivity. They are more or less dependent on intuition and non-verbal communication. This unarticulated dimension of engagement is always there, part and parcel of every clinical operation. Deliberately identifying and thoughtfully using the steps of the *conjunctive sequence* in clinical work gives form to this non-verbal aspect of treatment, making it accessible for deliberate clinician management.

Linking truing measures with clinical judgment

How much does physician self-discipline – for example, using the SO method, employing follow-up laboratory testing or psychometric assessment, or seeking a second opinion – count toward outcome (Moumjid *et al.*, 2007)? How does one know how much to emphasize a single truing measure or when to link several for obtaining the best results?

The answer is elusive and particular to each treatment. Collaboration meant everything in the work with Natalie; test results came first with Michael. The physician's goal, whatever truing measures are chosen to support it, needs to be to maximize the results of the treatment. The following truing methods particularly support this objective: (1) defining treatment goals in collaboration with the patient, (2) simultaneously identifying how outcome will be evaluated, and (3) progressively, and as formally as possible, assessing and recording the patient's progress.

As we consider the subject of optimizing outcome, we do well to recall the emotional, interactional, and organizational intricacies of an actual clinical process (also see Chapters 4 and 5). The final two chapters of this book will be devoted to our clinical methodology for organizing and dealing with these situations, focusing on the role of an MPCP treatment coordinator for managing clinically and operationally complex cases. Informing this approach is the debate between (1) the clinical certainty and verification that are inherent in evidence-based and empirically supported treatments, and (2) the place that intuition and clinical judgment inevitably play in our work (Mitchell, 1997; Mitchell & Aron, 1999; Downie & Mcnaughton, 2000; Wampold, 2001; Norcross, 2002; White & Stancombe, 2003).

Our task as physicians, then, is to keep an eye on the "operating characteristics" of the clinical problem at hand, maximizing true positives and minimizing the likelihood of getting wrong answers – false positives and false negatives. To do so we have to strive to methodically reduce the influence of subjectivity on our clinical decisions. Decisions made using clinical judgment alone, without empirical support, are basically guesses, albeit sometimes very good ones. Therefore, in addition to deliberately employing other truing measures, we always also need to find and stick with ways of identifying and monitoring our patient's progress and engaging that person as a collaborator.

Nathan

To test the value of combining truing measures with thoughtful clinical judgment, return to Nathan and his presumptive diagnosis of Parkinson's disease. At the onset of his illness, Nathan insisted that among his major problems were fear of aging and depression. His father had died at age 80, and Nathan was quickly approaching his 79th birthday. Parkinson's disease was clearly there. On physical examination there was some muscular rigidity, a mild but characteristic resting tremor, early postural instability, and detectable bradykinesia. True, Nathan's weakness, including its extent and distribution, was atypical, but that did not rule out Parkinson's disease. Also, Nathan's thinking and memory were unaffected and remained so until his death six years later.

According to his university-based physicians, Nathan's diagnosis was equivocal, most likely either a variant of *Parkinson's disease* or perhaps *multiple systems atrophy* predominantly involving his basal ganglia. The latter would help explain his accompanying gastrointestinal symptoms. Underpinning this set of opinions was a campaign by Nathan's daughter to promote the view that Nathan's condition was based entirely in systemic medical causes and was without a psychiatric component.

The clinical problem for me (SAF) was to sort between the stance taken by Nathan's physicians and daughter and Nathan's insistence that his symptoms were significantly related to anxiety and should be treated as such. At this point there was no agreement between participants in the case about the nature or even existence of a psychiatric disorder.

As part of this determination it was especially important to take a careful history. Nathan had convincing physical symptoms. However, differences from the usual presentation of Parkinson's disease were prominent. Nathan recounted a long history of gastrointestinal symptoms, weakness and muscles pains, and periodic episodes of disabling discouragement. Nathan also reported that he had been preparing for years to die in his late seventies, and was clear that he was satisfied with that prospect. As part of his personal preparation for the end of his life, however, he constantly had to buck his daughter's impatience with what she labeled his "passivity." Nathan simply wasn't interested in keeping himself physically fit and, like Solomon as he accepted his fate, he was progressively committed to shedding his usual social activities. He was willing to cooperate with his physicians and follow their medical recommendations, but that was it. Nathan was obdurate, sticking tenaciously to his own trajectory.

In an effort to sort between his psychiatric and systemic medical symptoms, Nathan agreed to a standard battery of cognitive and personality tests. Included were the MMPI-2, the Personality Assessment Inventory (PAI) (Morey, 2007), an abbreviated WAIS-R, and a Rorschach test.

The findings were quite useful in answering our questions about the nature of Nathan's illness. On the abbreviated WAIS-R, Nathan showed no areas of cognitive deficiency. The MMPI-2 did suggest that he was moderately depressed and clearly discouraged, although his depression was not severe enough to qualify as a Major Depressive Disorder (DSM-IV-TR 296.20). Of particular interest was an elevated psychosomatic score on the MMPI and PAI test batteries and the Rorschach. Especially informative was the finding on the Rorschach that Nathan's adjustment was adequate and that he was basically "realistic, able to face life challenges."

Strikingly, when several of these tests were repeated a year later, even the moderate depression was mostly gone, although Nathan's preoccupation with his body remained. Consistent with the assessment, Nathan said he had been only episodically depressed, while he was clearly troubled by his weakness and gastrointestinal symptoms since they were so unpleasant. Further, underscoring his view that he was fully competent to make judgments about his life were recent contacts between SAF and people who knew him well. According to them, Nathan was known and well respected in the community. He was an acclaimed musician. He was philanthropic. His children and grandchildren looked up to him.

Nathan said he was "sad" about not being able to please his daughter. Consequently, he agreed to comply with her insistence that he write his memoirs as a record of his life for his family. But, that was it. There were no clinical devices, no truing methods, left for making further clinical sense out of his "negativity." The only reasonable conclusion was that Nathan really did want to let go of life in a comfortable way and that he was perfectly content to do so. That was the criteria for success Nathan slated for his treatment.

Here is a sample of the dialogue between myself and Nathan. I had agreed to smoke cigars with Nathan during some of our sessions after he refused to engage in a sustained conversation under any other circumstance. Of course I was cognizant of the hazards of tobacco and understood the irony of smoking with a patient. However, in my opinion this situation called for an accommodation in order to make a meaningful exchange with Nathan possible.

SAF: "Nathan, what's your opinion (we are smoking cigars at the time), I want it straight."

Nathan: "Here it is, Steve. Everyone, and mostly my daughter, seems to be irritated by my being comfortable with dying. I need them all to get off the 'Nathan survival kick' and especially convince my daughter to do that. I've led a good life and really don't want to struggle with the rest of this. I can't even play the piano any more since my fingers don't move well. I'm less depressed, mainly stubborn at this point. Now let's smoke our cigars."

Using the understanding we had developed through our discussions and the test-based data we had collected, Nathan and I developed the following plan. (1) We would continue to work with Nathan's systemic medical problems. We had expert medical consultants on board, and I would work with and, as necessary, provide organization for his team of specialists. (2) I would speak with Nathan's daughter fairly regularly with the goal of helping her understand and abide by Nathan's wishes. (3) Nathan and I would continue our effort to unravel the psychological and existential issues fueling his discouragement, preparing the way for him to take greater management of his life as it moved into what he assumed were its final stages. To arrive at this sequence we made use of several truing operations mentioned thus far in this chapter, most particularly psychological assessment and clinical judgment based on the dialogue between Nathan and myself.

Neal

To further explore the value of collaboratively defining outcome measures we return to Neal. Notice the multiple, shifting sources of input that were involved in determining our treatment goals and monitoring Neal's progress. The initial work was difficult. Neal was unavailable for many months to engage in a heartfelt discussion about our work. Early on, Neal regarded psychiatric treatment as an imposition, an obligation that could usurp his age-associated insistence of doing life on his own. Psychometric assessment was helpful in providing direction but came late in the treatment. When they became available, the test-based findings about his ADHD and ways to manage it were especially helpful to us as we developed treatment goals.

In retrospect, what mattered most in facilitating my (SAF) early work with Neal and determining realistic treatment goals was my strategic decision to collaborate regularly with his parents. Of course, I guided them as well. For example, I recommended that apart from their collaboration with me, they be careful about criticism and interfere as little as possible with Neal's life. The requirement that Neal continue in treatment as a condition for their financial support was an exception to that rule.

The liaison with Neal's parents was especially useful in guiding my emotional connection with Neal. Neal was strikingly standoffish at the start of treatment, and I had to rely on my judgment that he privately craved an emotional connection to guide my clinical relationship with him. Without information from his parents, I had little certainty about whether my speculation was accurate or how to effect such a connection. With his parents' help I tracked Neal's progress, following the most important measures of his psychological functioning, including the nature of his social life, his moodiness, his comprom- ised ability to concentrate and work, his drinking, and his intention to return to college. On my own, I carefully followed treatment gains using an SO analysis which included the categories he and I successively identified for measuring his success.

More about the sequence of interpersonal experiences that guide the physician and patient: continuities and discontinuities that support treatment

Clinical progress – change desired by the physician and patient – is commonly disconnected chronologically from deliberately orchestrated clinical interven- tions. The type and quality of the connection between the physician and patient often radically alters at points surrounding change, with the reasons for those shifts frequently obscure. At each of these junctures, there is often a productive but frequently unanticipated and poorly understood discontinuity in the treatment process (the step in the *conjunctive sequence* referred to as "disruptions and repairs in the working relationship"). These points of change are often first appreciated only in retrospect. Certain steps in the *conjunctive sequence* including "controlled disorientation" combined with "mind clearing" and "leaps of inference" are especially implicated in creating these generative discontinuities (Frankel, S., 2007). The interpersonal impact of treatment is often greatest when the patient and physician seize these discontinuities strategically, as opportunities to deepen and further the treatment work.

There are also elusive interpersonally based treatment continuities; some that act as powerful supports for treatment. Reviewing the case illustration in Chapter 8 describing my work with Natalie, you may be impressed by how well we got along in spite of our differences and misunderstandings. In truth, our work was complicated, full of pitfalls. For example, Natalie and I did not initially agree about the alleged sexual molestations, with me being the more skeptical. In pursuing that subject Natalie had everything at stake, her probing potentially inciting her entire family's wrath. I had little to lose personally by engaging in our project, or at least so I thought. The point is that there were always so many issues with which to misunderstand each other and disagree about, so many ways we could have been at loggerheads. Yet, we never truly were. In effect, regardless of our differences, the affirmative continuities prevailed. Whatever else happened in the treatment, we both adhered to the same goal, the clarification and resolution of Natalie's personal distress and its association with the alleged childhood sexual molestations.

And the analogy in primary care medicine? Look simply at the continuities in my work with both Nathan and Keith. Both men were beset by systemic medical illnesses that monopolized their lives. Both had received advice from others that could have sabotaged their work with me. Neither ever hinted about terminating treatment.

Primary care physicians often do not to have the time in clinical practice to pay attention to the kind of interpersonal detail we describe. Nonetheless their work is affected, and usually supported, by the same interpersonal factors as that of psychiatrists. Of note, there is a flurry of writing by medical sociologists admonishing primary care physicians to pay close attention to and capitalize on these non-verbal aspects of patient–physician interaction (Frankel, R. *et al.*, 2003; Frankel, R. & Inui, 2006).

How much does each truing device contribute to clinical accuracy?

The answer to this question is tricky and is often influenced by factors only indirectly associated with the patient's presenting illness(es).

Here it makes sense to begin with primary care medicine. How many times have you heard of or seen a patient who was growing enfeebled or depressed and was relegated to the "functional" category by one or more physicians. Let's label that condition "chronic fatigue." Here we return to *Dorothy* from Chapter 3. She was given this diagnosis and died a few years later. On autopsy she proved to have disseminated cancer. Recall that she had given up hope of finding a cause for her symptoms months earlier and had stopped searching for an explanation.

What might a series of consultations with medical experts have offered her? In retrospect there were additional medical tests and diagnostic imaging procedures that would probably have revealed the nature of her disease. However, many of these assessments would have been expensive, and going through more workups, Dorothy alleged, would simply have tormented her. She said she was discouraged by her experience with the physicians who months earlier had, in effect, given up on her. So, whoever was to blame, Dorothy or her physicians, those tests and further workups were never done.

A second situation pertinent to our topic may be of interest. A patient comes in complaining of pain, in the area of his left shoulder, that is brought on by exertion. There are no other symptoms. On routine physical examination the internist hears a heart murmur. It may or may not be benign. The patient's last complete physical was three years ago and the murmur was not noted then. However, a cardiac stress test raises concerns and his physician orders an echocardiogram as well as coronary angiography.

It's just as she suspected. Two of the patient's coronary arteries are almost fully blocked. The diagnosis of coronary artery disease (CAD) is straightforward. But, even in this situation, getting a straight story from the patient and achieving compliance may be tricky. Among other measures, the physician tells the patient that he needs to stop smoking. The patient's reply is more equivocal. "I get it, Doc. I'll be fine and cut back my smoking." Notice, the patient, actually more honest than some, is not promising to stop smoking.

It's not only that the patient won't comply with medical recommendations; it's that more scrutiny would reveal that he believes that you, the physician, are exaggerating. His situation simply couldn't be so serious. In this case it is not the physician who needs truing in the service of establishing a diagnosis, it is the patient. If the physician in this situation needs data about anything, it is about the patient's psychology and how to understand it. This, of course, is a common clinical situation; one of many where the issue obstructing treatment is subsidiary to the systemic medical or psychiatric problem being targeted. Nonetheless, it is frequently necessary for a physician to grapple with, and often focus on, these sorts of problems as part of his or her ultimate responsibility as the patient's "doctor."

Primary care physicians might find it interesting to ask themselves how often they get an absolutely straight story from a patient. We would not be surprised if the answer was something like "are you kidding?" a code phrase for "rarely." People have all kinds of reasons, ranging from fear to ignorance, for not reporting straightforwardly on their medical condition, and each can block the way to adequate medical treatment.

We realize that we are confusing things by moving away from the strictly systemic medical or psychiatric aspects of the situations we are describing. But, that is the way it is with clinical work. There are always unexpected deviations and detours that come up, and these can be introduced from just about any source, including the patient's personal life. In the example just given, laboratory tests and diagnostic imaging were unequivocally helpful for the physician as she attempted to make a diagnosis. However, when the patient heard about the results, the news had the paradoxical effect of inflaming his doubts about the physician's opinions. His reaction was unrelated to the medical issue at hand and temporarily became the most profound influence on the near-term course of the treatment.

Return to the topic of this section, "How much does each truing device contribute to clinical accuracy?" The truing measures available to us are, of course, each quite useful. Nonetheless, it would be hard to put a number on the relative importance of any one of these. Each intersects with a particular case differently, potentially yielding divergent categories of information. And no one can predict or fully account for the idiosyncrasies and surprises that so often characterize and influence the clinical process, especially in work with complex cases.

Accountability: truing (honesty) required by patients

The accusation from a patient I (SAF) saw this morning keeps resounding in my brain as I work on this chapter. He wondered where I got the "audacity to charge such high fees," when as a psychiatrist all I do is "sit around and talk." How did I know that what I do actually works? Did I have statistics? Here, of course, is where the accountability, the evidence that supports claims a physician makes about his or her clinical work, comes in.

This patient's diatribe is reminiscent of Marty's, who unrelentingly accused me (SAF) of being unreasonable in charging him for a missed appointment (Chapter 8). Accountability with *Marty* might have benefitted from some of the following measures. Using them would probably have improved my clinical assessment of him and helped me better understand what kind of response Marty needed from me.

(1) I might have enlisted a consultant to help me sort out the validity of his allegation that I was being punitive by insisting he pay for a missed session. In truth, I was unable to recognize my irritation with him; nor was I aware of its source in his continual criticism of me.

(2) It might have helped had I obtained a psychometric assessment early in that case, since it almost certainly would have revealed that Marty harbored a propensity for paranoia that was not usually apparent from the surface.

(3) My impression of Marty actually benefitted from an arranged encounter with him outside my office: an experience challenging the validity of my

office-based clinical impression. In this situation, at his request, I met him for an appointment at a coffee shop.

(4) Speaking with family members or other collateral informants might accomplish something similar to an extra-office encounter by providing a comparison view of the patient.

(5) Less problematic than speaking with collateral informants is contacting outside sources for information, particularly other physicians who have treated the patient.

Move again to Keith and Nathan and the personal accountability patients often need from their physicians. Neither Keith nor Nathan would have worked productively with me (SAF) had I been blandly technical with them about their systemic medical and psychiatric conditions. Neither would have omitted an agreeable, albeit straightforward, relationship with his physicians from his criteria for satisfactory treatment. In that respect, both men counted on me to understand their fears, explain their medical and psychological illness to them as well as their families, and clarify medical developments as they came up. In those particular cases the other treating physicians were stuck, either unable or unwilling to take a definitively helpful stance. In Nathan's situation the diagnosis was frustratingly elusive; in Keith's the primary physician was unwilling to put Keith's agenda before his own.

Precision in clinical work revisited

In this chapter we have pitted the neatness of tests and examinations against the less organized tapestry of clinical judgment. Clinical judgment is a response to the events in practice, dictating on-the-spot ways to deal with them. Truing measures, brought in as the case moves on, keep the clinical process focused on the problems for which the patient came to treatment. These issues are incorporated into treatment goals and outcome measures, revised periodically throughout the treatment.

Indeed, the clinical process is complicated. It is neither amenable to objectification nor safely guided by intuition. The physician needs to be a good technician, able to follow the progress of the case with reasonable accuracy. He or she needs equally to be engaged in the work as a human being interacting with another human being. In the first role the physician feels and acts like a scientist. In the second, he or she faces the uncertainties of his or her craft and the true interpersonal complexity of the clinical challenge. As physicians, truing measures are our defense against chaos. We can usually do well with them, so long as we are able to tolerate the uncertainties that, nonetheless, remain after using them.

However, this is a traditional two-person practice model. It reflects clinical reality when only the physician and the patient are interacting. But, when the number of specialists required to address the patient's problems multiplies, the administrative structure changes. In these situations a person in the role of a treatment coordinator, an MPCP, can, and often should, be added to the treatment configuration. Earlier in the book we designated this additional structural dimension of the treatment, comprised of the treatment coordinator and his or her responsibilities, "Level 2." The clinical situation is then transformed so that it involves multiple participants, each one with his or her own technical capabilities, requirements, and personality. Further, these people interact, adding the psychology of their relationships, its impact on the patient and the treatment outcome, to the influences in the treatment.

With Alan it was never a matter of his immunologists treating his systemic medical problems by themselves, or SAF alone dealing with his psychiatric illness. All these specialists interacted, and the nature and quality of their interaction fundamentally impacted the case. In fact, it was their failure to pull together as a cooperating treatment team that was so problematic. Also, Alan's wife always threatened to bring her issues back onto the scene, potentially upsetting the harmony of Alan's work with SAF. And the result? The consequence of failing to effect a viable, cooperating treatment team? You already know it. Alan never received his bone marrow transplant.

More on truing and its application at the level of the MPCP in Chapter 10.

10

Managing complex treatments: the medical–psychiatric coordinating physician

Clinical work can seem reasonably straightforward when reduced to its fundamentals in an EBT or EST algorithm. Unfortunately, what gets lost here is the patient as a non-linear, feeling and reacting human being. In contrast, limiting clinical work to its most subjective activity – clinical judgment – is equally likely to produce aberrant results. Additional complications are introduced when the patient's presentation is complex, includes co-morbid conditions involving psychiatric and systemic medical illnesses, and requires the attention of a multispecialty treatment team. In this chapter we continue to present our approach to working with this category of patient, further describing the MPCP model for organizing and optimizing their care. Of note, in Chapter 1 we suggest a clinical role parallel to that of the MPCP when psychiatric co-morbidity is not in evidence. In that case leadership of the treatment team can be accorded to a PCP, who becomes a *Coordinating Physician* and takes on duties analogous to those of the MPCP.

In Chapters 2 and 9 we made the point that there aren't many clinical situations that, when looked at closely, consist of only two people. Left out of the traditional physician–patient model are other physicians and allied healthcare professionals, as well as the omnipresent, but often silent, influencers of treatment, including the patient's spouse, children, parents, boss, and culture. We believe the medical–psychiatric coordinating physician (MPCP) model of care represents a realistic expansion of the standard two-person treatment model, encompassing this reality. Psychiatric specialization for this coordinating role is called for when the case includes co-morbidity dominated by psychopathology. Recall from Chapter 1 that we designated the subgroup of patients for whom this type and level of care is especially appropriate: *psychiatrically co-morbid, management-intensive, complex patients.*

Innovation and the MPCP

There is no fixed protocol for the work of the MPCP. Even our truing measures may prove anemic when clinical issues are pressing and the case is burdened by complexities. An acclaimed pianist, a realist about life, Nathan was nonetheless clear that his physicians were "off-base." Nathan's physicians were top-notch, technically experienced, and attentive; experts in neurological diseases including variants of Parkinson's disease. His office-based internist was proactive about Nathan's systemic medical needs. But, Nathan, who was ordinarily agreeable with physicians, had his own ideas about these matters, and progressively went "on strike," refusing to cooperate with treatment.

Nathan's medical center physicians also did a good job of following his disease. But there were four of them, and after the beginning of treatment, they seemed to talk with one another only when there was a crisis or a formal request for a consultation. Working with Nathan through the maze of his and his physicians' opinions, and the interpersonal issues posed by Nathan's and his daughter's disagreement, required a physician treatment coordinator: an MPCP.

The MPCP's therapeutic role

It would, of course, be good to ask whether the role taken by the MPCP *itself* enhances treatment. Components of treatment are already being provided by other professionals. On a treatment team there is always a primary care physician and often, as in Nathan's case, several physician specialists. In addition to the patient, there are also frequently family members who join with the team as collaborators.

And, yet, judging by our clinical experience, the whole in an MPCP-led treatment is distinctly greater than the sum of its parts. It is our impression that *introducing an MPCP into a complex treatment enhances its power and not just its organization.* That is, the role of the MPCP itself seems to have therapeutic impact resulting in part from the vision, the framework, and the overall coherence it provides. The MPCP also needs to be accountable for results and cognizant of the mechanisms through which these are occurring, continually assessing whether the treatment is going according to plan. It also usually matters to the patient and family that the MPCP is independently available to discuss the treatment, its technicalities, and how well it is working. Consistently, the MPCP actually needs to have the mind-set that he or she is not just managing a complex treatment, but, in effect, is providing a therapeutic function for the patient's entire clinical system.

How the MPCP affects the direction of the treatment

In each of the following cases SAF was the MPCP, in charge of managing the treatment team. In Nathan's case the team consisted of his internist, neurologist, and several other consulting specialists. For Larry, who you will meet in a moment, in addition to SAF who prescribed psychotropic medication for ADHD and mood stabilization, there was an internist, a rheumatologist who treated Larry's recurrent idiopathic autoimmune hemolytic anemia, two psychologists who at different times administered personality and neuropsychological assessment, and a personal assistant with training in learning disabilities who helped Larry organize his life.

In the two vignettes below, SAF needed to respond to a crisis before he was able to consult with team members. Immediate action was required to avert a personal crisis for both patients and prevent the likely destruction of the treatment. The MPCP is frequently called upon to take this kind of unilateral stance. Subsequently, his or her decision and future clinical strategy is discussed with the other team members. Incidentally, this kind of intervention represents the application on the MPCP level of the "leap of inference" described in Chapter 8 as one component of the "conjunctive sequence" described there.

Nathan

Let's say a patient has an acquaintance who suddenly begins to talk against you, his or her physician. That, in fact, is what started to happen with Nathan's daughter. She alleged that it was me, SAF, who was responsible for Nathan's loss of interest in finding a cure for his condition. In fact, it was she who did not accept that Nathan's convictions about his life coming to an end might be realistic. Her insinuation was that if I, SAF, was just more upbeat in my work with him, Nathan's condition might improve and he might even be cured. She had been supportive of treatment to that point. The psychological mechanism underlying her dramatic shift is technically called "splitting" (Grotstein, 1981; Ogden, 1982). This term refers to a way people attempt to resolve a personal dilemma through demonizing a previously idealized figure.

Nathan's daughter's shift was not an incidental development for Nathan, who already felt quite unsupported in his desire for a relatively peaceful exit from life. Actually, apart from me, no one seemed particularly ready to support Nathan's preference. A conventional clinical stance in dealing with the disagreement between Nathan and his daughter would have been to let them work their problems out by themselves and simply attend to Nathan's systemic medical and psychiatric illness. My judgment, however, was that, if Nathan was not going to crash into utter despair, he needed someone to advocate for him. As a result, I took on two direct therapeutic roles in addition to my coordinating position as MPCP. The first was as Nathan's individual psychotherapist and the second as mediator to the relationship between Nathan and his daughter. During this time I was in touch with all team members, particularly Nathan's internist. I needed to make sure they would cooperate with me and not join with Nathan's daughter's effort to bypass his needs and wishes.

In taking this stance with Nathan and his daughter, I wanted to avert an outcome similar to Keith's when he lost all personal agency during his convoluted medical odyssey. In this regard, I also thought about how Alan's wife had chronically undermined him as he attempted to enjoy the last months of his life.

Larry

Similar family issues were raised in the work with Larry. Larry was 40 years old when he entered treatment, and had been divorced for two years. Diagnostically, he suffered from a Depressive Disorder (DSM-IV-TR 311, Depressive Disorder Not Otherwise Specified), severe ADHD, and a relatively independent derangement involving his executive functions. He had been forced twice to drop out of an "on-line" law school because of the erratic nature of his performance.

Larry was originally referred to SAF by his neurologist and primary care physician after his disorganization caused him to lose several jobs, as well as his marriage, and to take risks that twice landed him in jail. He also had developed a gambling addiction that was in part sustained by his inability to keep track of his finances. Larry's mother was also very much in the picture since one of Larry's objectives for treatment was to address his disordered relationship with his mother and his siblings. Both she and Larry were also concerned about the impact of Larry's damaged self-esteem on the way he conducted his life and his impaired motivation for personal change – problem areas that they assumed were linked to Larry's father's alcoholism and abusiveness during Larry's childhood.

As background, Larry was always in turmoil. Typically, he'd forget to renew his driver's license, neglect to collect rent checks for a building in which he shared ownership, or overdraw his bank account. More troubling, when he went to Southern California to visit his mother he would typically end up in Las Vegas for a few weeks, gamble away his money, and not return to take care of business or attend appointments.

The "acquaintance" in this case, Larry's ex-wife, still had a great deal of influence with him. At this point she was apparently feeling competitive with me, SAF, for Larry's loyalty and was compelled to insinuate herself into his treatment. She began by haranguing Larry, saying that "psychiatry induces people to be lazy thinkers." Larry had been devastated by her decision to terminate their marriage two years earlier. He was still desperate to reengage her, and soon began to take the message of her tirades seriously.

In a situation of this sort, as the treating psychiatrist, you would be ill-advised to assume that such an incursion would be inconsequential for a treatment that Larry so clearly required. As his psychiatrist you could have attempted to take a conventional path and explored the development with Larry, focusing on his anxieties and his ex-wife's motivations. On the contrary, you might have reasoned, as I did, that confronting him with the ostensible maliciousness of his ex-wife's behavior might not be powerful enough to influence him to be more self-protective and, in addition, might create a loyalty conflict for him. The threat to our hard-won treatment alliance was acute. I was certain of that. We needed a good strategy, and we needed it fast.

Returning to my role as MPCP, I had to make sure the others who were working with us, especially Larry's mother who had a great deal of influence with him, would join with my strategy. To this end, their support was quickly mobilized.

What to do about EBT and EST protocols in this situation? At that juncture we were no longer primarily treating Larry's depression, ADHD, and executive function impairment. As I saw it, what Larry needed most at that moment was a trusted ally, someone whose voice could be heard above his ex-wife's. This person would have to take responsibility for pulling together the disparate pieces of Larry's faltering life. He or she would have to show him, in a way more convincing than the ex-wife, that they had a superior plan for dealing with his problems and confidence in his capabilities. You heard us right. We did not say that person needed to help him pull his faltering life together. We said, perhaps somewhat surprisingly, that this person would have to take responsibility for pulling the pieces of his faltering life together.

Was it appropriate for me to provide such a function? If the answer is "yes," what does that stance have to do with principles of psychotherapy, which traditionally hold that the clinician catalyzes change rather than becoming embroiled in creating it? By the way, Nathan, early in his work with me (SAF), had similar requirements as he grappled with inexplicable weakness in his lower extremities and with bowel problems. In that situation the factor primarily impeding treatment was discouragement, preventing Nathan from getting and following the medical help he needed. I had to come in as Nathan's advocate, providing advice and guidance for him. In that role, in order to create a personal bond with him, I seized on "kibitzing." That was the term that Nathan used to refer to a playful, half-serious conversation with an underlying, meaningful philosophical theme. The connection that was enabled in this way seemed to bring Nathan back to life and into a cooperative frame of mind.

Commentary

In these two pressing situations no team member other than myself, the MPCP, had the kind of perspective and leverage required for deciding to take a pre-emptive stand. While I was the personal psychiatrist for both Nathan and Larry, in acting unilaterally as MPCP I was also choosing a course of action for the team. In Nathan's case, for example, in addition to my psychotherapeutic role, I had the delicate responsibility of enlisting Nathan's daughter as well as the team members to join with my revised strategy.

Both situations, Larry's and Nathan's, called for quick, strategic thinking and a rapid shift in clinical posture until the halted treatment could get off the ground again. In each case, the team members needed to be mobilized to support the MPCP's leadership. There was plenty of evidence in each situation to support my assuming a personally involved, "real" role with the patient. Confirmation of the wisdom of this choice came from collaboration with the patient as well as with team members; physician self-reflection using an SO analysis; and, in Nathan's case, psychological assessment.

The SO analysis for Nathan suggested that he was actually happiest when allowed to indulge in his chosen involutional course: curled up by himself in bed, while reviewing his life and contemplating its end. The "self" aspect for him was paradoxically one of satisfaction with the course he had chosen for himself. In the "other" dimension people were portrayed as potentially interfering with his sense of tranquility. "Self with other" almost didn't exist since Nathan mostly wanted to be left alone. In his mind a psychiatric treatment session mainly ran its course after a good philosophical discussion and, in some cases, a cigar.

As noted, it was important in both situations that members of the treatment team be quickly brought along to support the revised strategies. As MPCP I needed to enlist them and keep them informed until the crisis abated. In Nathan's case, one team member, Nathan's daughter, was dissident, and organizing the other team members to initially take a stance different from hers required a good deal of diplomacy. In that situation my stance as MPCP created a personal conflict for the internist on the team since he had worked closely with Nathan's daughter for years. Several long phone calls were necessary before he felt comfortable with the new strategy.

More on the MPCP's clinical judgment: tricks of the trade

In this chapter thus far we have discussed the therapeutic importance of the MPCP's role and the place of the MPCP in rapidly modifying team strategy in a crisis. Here we turn to the subject of how the patient's initial complaints may shift or evolve as a result of unexpected developments, calling for a modified treatment plan.

With Nathan, the breakthrough in my (SAF's) ability to work with him happened when I discovered his love for cigars. His daughter hated Nathan's cigar smoking, and Nathan experienced her attitude as intended to spoil this last vestige of pleasure in his progressively miserable life. As described in Chapter 9, the strategy for effective clinical work with him at this point became quite obvious and was not very technical. I needed Nathan to take my clinical advice to heart. So, since in this case a cigar would not be "just a cigar" but rather a therapeutic device, I offered to smoke cigars with him as we talked. As you know, he was delighted by this prospect and joined up with me. Shortly thereafter, as Nathan came to trust me, he reiterated his permission for me to deal with his daughter as well as provide organization for his other physicians.

And Larry? Indeed he was distracted by his ex-wife in the incident recounted earlier. To understand that event, recall the profound influence on his life of his ADHD and executive function impairment. He was a bright, lovely guy who couldn't stay a straight course without guidance and medication. My follow-up strategy, after the ex-wife crisis was resolved, squarely addressed the disorganization of his life. At about that point, his mother became convinced enough of the potential value of neuropsychological testing to agree to provide part of the financial support for it. Larry's insurance company had previously rejected several requests for this level of psychometric assessment. The information the assessment provided turned out to be monumental since, together with electro-encephalographic information, it introduced an entirely new factor into the diagnostic picture. Unlike the findings of personality assessment two years previously, this more exacting test battery, together with a neurological workup, suggested complex partial seizures[1] (ICD-10-CM G40.20, Partial Complex Seizures) as part of the explanation for Larry's "mood swings" and instability.

Clinical accuracy

Clinical accuracy, accounting for the independent variables, the "Xs" we talked about in Chapter 2, is a topic that has been with us throughout this book. It is appropriate for us to return to it before moving onward. We begin again with a single proposition: clinical perfection is an admirable, necessary, but never fully reachable, goal. There are always independent variables that remain unaccounted for and which affect clinical accuracy. Sometimes results are more dependable and sometimes less so. Inability to achieve treatment goals is rarely explained by physician failure alone. Clinical work just has its limitations. There is no clinical process that is not plagued by subjectivity (Abelson, 1985; Aron, 1991, 1992; Renik, 1993; Tanenbaum, 1993; Watson & Rennie, 1994) and is entirely reliable over time. Closing the gap, however, improving the precision of our work as we attempt to control for the variance introduced by these independent variables, are our truing measures.

Our case examples illustrate how this process works. For Nathan the SO analysis alluded to above provided data for me (SAF) to come up with a strategy that helped him accept the medical care he required. Nathan's disillusionment with life, however, had to be understood and acknowledged first. Only then would he be willing to think about and discuss medical issues in a way that "had teeth." As I got to understand Nathan, I had to make it clear that I was on his side, supporting his wishes for managing the last phase of his life. I then had to find a personal vehicle – in this case "kibitzing" and smoking a cigar – to buttress that process. The work was eventually made even more substantial by psychological test findings that confirmed the earnestness of Nathan's stated desire to finish his life in his own way.

For Neal a key source of truing was input from his parents, and, ultimately even more important, collaborative feedback from Neal as he probed to see how personally committed I was to him. Personality and neuropsychological assessment came relatively late in the process.

Using our case examples it becomes obvious that the same truing devices may not be equally useful in each treatment. With Solomon, essential categories of information would have been missing if some treatment sessions hadn't been

---

[1] Also designated "psychomotor" or "temporal lobe" epilepsy.

conducted at his apartment. These meetings allowed me to observe the progress or deterioration of Solomon's personal habits, providing a check on his son's and daughter-in-law's allegations that his inattention to personal hygiene was jeopardizing his health. From there, one of the most revealing truing devices was psychometric assessment. While neuropsychological assessment had confirmed his intact cognitive status, personality assessment underscored my suspicion that Solomon's emotional resilience, expressed mainly as ostensible withdrawal from social relationships, had initially been misinterpreted as depression. For Neal, truing included the unusual arrangement for collaborative feedback with his parents.

Both Neal's and Solomon's treatments involved a treatment team. That team in Solomon's case included an internist, immunologist, dermatologist, nutritionist, Solomon's family as collaborators, and SAF as the psychiatrist. Neal's team was comprised of a neurologist, neuropsychologist, a psychologist who carried out CBT sessions, his parents as active collaborators, and SAF.

The MPCP and Level 2 truing

The truing devices mentioned in the preceding paragraphs are applicable for directing and monitoring dyadic physician–patient interactions. These are the activities we classified as constituting "Level 1" of the clinical process. This system of classification was introduced in Chapter 1 and further elaborated in Chapter 8. "Level 2," in contrast, refers to the assortment of people and care delivery systems involved in a complex case and therefore to the coordinating work of the MPCP. Truing on this clinical level focuses on outcome measures, with the maintenance of overall treatment progress as its clinical objective.

To carry out his or her clinical role the MPCP needs to be conversant with all technical topics relevant to the case, including issues that are likely to come up in the communication with and between team members, as well as with outside agencies and consultants. Some areas of required familiarity follow. (1) First, the MPCP needs to understand the pathophysiology of the patient's illness(es). For example, SAF needed to be knowledgeable about Parkinson's disease with Nathan, scleroderma and osteoarthritis with Solomon, and assorted systemic medical complaints in Neal's case. (2) Second, for the sake of credibility with them, the MPCP needs to have a solid understanding of each team member's specialty. (3) Third, the MPCP in the role as treatment coordinator also has to account for each team member's psychology as it impacts the team. This requirement will be illustrated later in this chapter using Nathan's experience with the medical-center-based physicians, who initially failed to acknowledge the importance to the case of Nathan's internist and SAF, both based outside of the university. (4) Finally, truing at the MPCP level is maintained by intermittent verbal or written reports from each team member to the MPCP and then status reports from the MPCP to team members.

The MPCP also continually gathers information needed to strategize the work of the team. The truing goal here is to assure that the team's work is efficient and its objectives well chosen. Experience in conflict resolution is required for the MPCP to manage disagreements among team members, as well as the patient and family as they affect treatment. Keeping Nathan's wife and internist, or Solomon's son and daughter-in-law, in the clinical fold are examples. Also, along with his or her other roles, the MPCP communicates with the patient and often the patient's family in order to be current about their needs and attitudes, as well as to keep them in touch with clinical developments. In this role the MPCP is a personal resource for them.

The limits of certainty: Hilary

So, what is the bottom line in how a physician operating independently or as MPCP can reliably find his or her way? This section is a bit of a departure from our goal of developing a comprehensive model for structuring a complex treatment, but we think it is pertinent and revealing.

Recently my (SAF) wife and I needed to find a cardiovascular surgeon for my 28-year-old stepdaughter, Hilary. She had a badly damaged mitral valve that now was implicated in the rapid deterioration in her cardiac functioning. The situation was inexpressibly frightening for my wife, myself, and most assuredly for my stepdaughter. Nonetheless, the challenge of finding the right surgeon at first seemed straightforward. Just choose the person with the best reputation. Frequently in surgery, personality and bedside manner hardly count at all.

Here is how it went, however. With myself as a psychiatrist and my wife a neuropsychologist, we had a good medical background and excellent professional connections on our side. We acquainted ourselves with the medical literature. Of the six eminent surgeons with whom we initially met, three said Hilary could wait for months or even years before having surgery. The other three said the surgery needed to be done immediately, with emphasis on the word "immediately." All six seemed completely sure of themselves. Each had cogent reasons for his or her apparently non-negotiable position.

During the course of these meetings we became aware that the anatomy and physiology of Hilary's cardiac lesions were unusual. Confused and frightened, we arranged to have more medical tests scheduled: mainly echocardiograms taken from different anatomical positions and under a variety of test conditions. The results were equivocal: her left ventricle was somewhat enlarged, ejection fraction compromised, and her cardiovascular dynamics were abnormal with exercise.

It was time to turn again to the medical literature. We read over three hundred articles and multiple book chapters. One thing we were learning was how opinionated experts can become about their specialty area. Each surgeon we visited had unparalleled training and a vast amount of experience. All six had a definite position about whether my stepdaughter was a candidate for either repair or replacement of her badly distorted valve and when the operation should occur. Each claimed to have excellent statistics for their mitral valve operations.

However, no matter how many times we requested it, outcome data – each one's success in correctly diagnosing and operating on this esoteric type of mitral valve lesion – never was fully available. Also, the challenge of sorting among surgeons was made even harder by the fact that the surgeons used different language to describe their work in this area; some called it "mitral valve replacement and repair," some limited their list to "complex mitral valve repairs," and only one or two categorized this operation under what turned out to be its technically correct surgical and diagnostic heading, repair and replacement of a Barlow's (syndrome) valve.

Every time we thought we were coming to the end of our painstaking search, we hit a wall of disagreement among surgeons or lack of clarity in how they represented their work and results. So, where was the certainty for which we were searching? We had chosen some of the best surgeons in the world. We had multiple interviews with each. Most of them were quite gracious, and all did their best to address our questions. We had read more literature than even some of the surgeons. Since each surgeon unequivocally believed in his or her findings and opinion, here, then, in bright lights are the limits bounding physician certainty in systemic medicine, even in surgery.

By making this statement we do not mean to imply that the reading we did and our discussions with experts, in effect the truing devices we employed, were not useful. Disciplining ourselves in these ways was, in fact, very orienting. Ultimately, we indeed were in a much better position to choose among technical procedures and surgeons. But certainty? Sadly, there did not seem to be any such thing available to us. In the end, regardless of how much technical information we had amassed, our decision had to be guided in part by our gut feelings about the surgeons we interviewed.

Return now to clinical work. Since we are convinced that truing devices improve the accuracy of our work, we still need to ask how much each one contributes. What information can guide us as we try to determine which are likely to be most useful and under what clinical circumstances? Ultimately how much better is one approach to a clinical problem than another? The answer, unfortunately, is that "hard," published research data about this issue generally come from group studies and may not be applicable to individuals for whose treatment these guides are used. While it may be tempting to extrapolate the findings of population studies to individuals, one needs to be cautious about doing that. A reasonable assumption, then, is that the power of individual truing measures is ultimately case specific. Decisions about which truing measures to rely upon in a particular case are in part empirical, should be undertaken when developing and revising a treatment plan, and are likely to be modified as treatment progresses.

Move then to the MPCP as coordinator in complex cases. The MPCP needs to evaluate data from diverse sources. In Hilary's case, I as a physician, and my wife as a neuropsychologist, together her "unofficial MPCPs," had to be knowledgeable when we spoke with cardiologists, cardiovascular surgeons, and radiologists. We also needed to have grasped the relevant medical literature and assimilated the recommendations of experts without either idealizing the reported findings or getting lost in extraneous detail.

To be most effective, therefore, a physician functioning as a MPCP should be specifically trained for that role. Especially with the clinical group we uniquely target for MPCP care – *psychiatrically co-morbid, management-intensive, complex patients* – he or she needs to be part each of a psychiatrist, primary care physician, psychologist, and family systems expert, as well as conversant with whatever other specialties are pertinent to a particular case. These capabilities, of course, are matched by the actual involvement of appropriate medical specialists. Enforcing this point, it is hard to imagine my wife and I having successfully steered Hilary's treatment in the absence of an actual MPCP without the benefit of our strong backgrounds in medicine and biology.

Results!

We are left with the question of how a physician knows a procedure is succeeding. Here is where monitoring progress comes in, bringing with it some additional challenges. In the following section, references to the treatment monitoring responsibility of the individual physician and MPCP are interchangeable.

For Nathan, ironically, outcome initially had to be judged mainly according to his level of depression and his satisfaction that his insistence on living out his life in his own way was being respected, not primarily by the symptomatic management of his neurological condition. The systemic medical focus was on his Parkinson's disease and his growing weakness and debilitation. He, instead, seemed far less invested in his health and survival than in his desire to withdraw peacefully from life, while still assuaging his daughter. As a reminder, in most complex clinical cases, the psychiatric and systemic medical are intertwined. With Nathan we did not have real hope of touching the systemic issues without paying major attention to the psychiatric.

Probing to see whether progress was occurring in Larry's case created another set of challenges, and generated new findings as well as modified outcome criteria. A year before the ex-wife challenge, Larry had a repeat battery of personality tests. At that time he could not afford to pay for a test battery that included neuropsychological assessment. According to those tests, Larry was less depressed and more capable of planning and task execution, making him appear ready to return to law school. It looked like the pain of his divorce was behind him. In addition to the test findings, indications of clinical success were flashing "green." However, his ex-wife's incursion a year or so later was such a shock that it seriously unbalanced him and flew in the face of our conviction about Larry's resilience.

It is important to note in this discussion that we are not judging clinical progress by reference to population statistics. Instead, we are working according to the model of "single-subject research" (Kazdin, 1998; McMillan, 2004). Each case is its own "research project." When, as in Larry's case, there is functional regression, it needs to be explained by reference to truing measures applicable to that particular patient. In Larry's case these measures included serial psychological, personality and neuropsychological, assessments. In sequence, hypotheses about the patient's psychopathology and prognosis need to be revised in accordance with new truing information and indications of clinical progress.

In Larry's situation, our original formulation and impression of his prognosis were incomplete and had not accounted for his intense loneliness and desire to redo the trauma of the divorce. His lingering hope was that repair of his failed marriage was possible. And, so, testing or not, and in spite of our best efforts, we got it wrong. As we discovered, required of us was recognition that key factors influencing Larry's personal adjustment had changed. We needed to be flexible enough to revise our clinical formulation and modify our outcome criteria to include his insufficient capacity to manage loss.

Additionally, the intensity and abruptness of Larry's reaction to his ex-wife's intrusion ultimately tipped us off that something further might be missing from the test findings and case formulation. At that point Larry's mother's financial help had been secured, and we were fortunate enough to be able to arrange for a neuropsychological test battery and an additional neurological assessment. For the first time, as a result of this assessment and electroencephalographic information, we had evidence suggesting that, along with his ADHD and executive dysfunction problems, complex partial epileptic seizures were probably implicated in explaining Larry's erratic behavior. Once again, for a third time, the formulation for this case needed to be modified.

Progress and outcome

Principles applicable to the monitoring of clinical progress and illustrated by these two examples include the following.
(1) Each case is its own research project. According to the principle of single-subject research (Kazdin, 1998; McMillan, 2004), the subject is his or her own control for judging the efficacy of the clinical work.
(2) Outcome criteria are different for each case. They are established at the outset of treatment and are repeatedly revised as treatment progresses. As in Larry's case, new categories may be added over time. These criteria are originally defined according to the problems that brought the patient to treatment, and revised in collaboration with the patient as time goes on.
(3) The patient and physician need to be aware that there is nothing particularly enduring about the outcome criteria initially adopted for a case. These measures often shift as treatment progresses and new clinical issues are identified. Required is that these criteria be clearly defined and agreed upon

by the patient and physician. It is often useful to commit them to writing so both physician and patient are clear about and assisted in following them.

(4) Repeat clinical examinations and testing, psychiatric and systemic medical, may be helpful in following progress and confirming that the outcome criteria remain appropriate and are being met.

A comprehensive treatment protocol and the medical–psychiatric coordinating physician

It bears repeating that no diagnosis or treatment plan is complete without all implicated factors being considered. In addition to the patient's systemic medical and psychiatric status, there are the patient's and family's real-life challenges. Added may be cultural issues and their influence on how inclined the patient and family are to cooperate with treatment.

Genetic and other biological considerations may influence treatment choices and methods. Medical specialists, including those who can consult on matters with which the other physicians involved in the case or the MPCP are not familiar, or allied health professionals such as a learning disabilities expert or nutritionist, may be needed if the case is to be fully understood and adequately managed. The patient's resources may place a cap on the extent and duration of treatment. Where insurance reimbursement is part of the picture, the choice of experts and procedures may be limited, at times making it necessary to locate and coordinate with specialists for whose services a patient needs to pay out of pocket.

Ideally, a primary care physician should be able to think comprehensively enough to take this entire range of contributing factors into consideration. However, this requirement is quite unrealistic given the demands it would make on that physician's time and focus. Here, then, is where the MPCP comes in. That role is designed to encompass care for complex patients, in particular those with psychiatric co-morbidity, while at the same time tracking progress and troubleshooting problems as they develop, including team-related difficulties.

Considering this distinction in roles, we believe the MPCP designation could eventually qualify as a separate medical subspecialization and, in particular, a psychiatric subspecialization when patients with psychiatric co-morbidity are predominantly involved. As you know, the MPCP almost always works on at least two levels. To reiterate, on Level 1 that person may function as a treating physician. In this role he or she uses standard truing measures to keep his or her part of the treatment on track. On Level 2, as strategist-coordinator for the treatment team, the MPCP uses outcome measures to provide direction for the treatment team. These criteria are collaboratively set and revised by the MPCP in collaboration with the patient and team members. The assortment of truing and outcome measures that prove most useful hold for a single case only and may not to be germane to other cases. As a reminder, responsibility on the level of team administration, MPCP Level 2, also is stratified. It consists of (1) soliciting and dealing with communication from and with team members, and (2) using this information to modify the treatment plan as well as negotiate compromises when there is lack of agreement among team members.

The realities

Details of Nathan's case beyond those already given should help illustrate the contrast between the ideal and real in clinical work, the latter being the complicated field in which the clinician always functions and the field of operation for all MPCP-led treatments.

Nathan's primary physician, a superb general practitioner, was sure that Nathan had a neurological illness, a variant of Parkinson's disease. However, as you know, its manifestations were not typical. By that point Nathan had already developed fecal incontinence along with his weakness. Because of the challenge of managing the incontinence and the associated humiliation, Nathan progressively withdrew. Frustrated and dismayed, Nathan's daughter independently arranged for a comprehensive medical evaluation at a well-known multidisciplinary clinic. Recall that the daughter disagreed with the diagnostic opinions and management recommendations of virtually everyone who, like Nathan, believed that psychiatric issues were implicated in Nathan's deteriorating condition. Nathan's primary care physician, who was thoughtful but not very psychiatrically oriented, overlooked the potential emotional impact on Nathan of his acceding to Nathan's daughter's insistence on the extensive evaluation without gaining Nathan's heartfelt assent. Nathan's acquiescence to their decision was weak and never tested for its authenticity by either the daughter or the PCP.

After a week of medical testing and the growing realization that Nathan's systemic medical symptoms didn't entirely make sense to them, the physicians at that clinic ordered a psychiatric consultation. The local psychosomatic medicine psychiatrist visited on the same day and prescribed aripiprazole 10 mg, assuming that the required fix involved the containment of Nathan's uncontrolled anxiety. No plan was made for the consultant to return. Note the repeated shifts between a systemic medical and psychiatric focus here and throughout this portion of the case description. Unexpectedly, within a few weeks Nathan's fatalism, bowel symptoms, and depression all peaked. At this point, Nathan stopped talking to virtually everyone.

On Nathan's return home after two weeks, a similar sequence repeated itself at the local university medical center. Included again were visits from a psychosomatic medicine psychiatrist, this time called in because of both Nathan's anxiety and obvious despondency. By then Nathan's primary care physician was for the most part out of the picture. The university-based physicians conferred among themselves about Nathan's medical management but were too busy to include physicians associated with the case who were located outside the medical center. Also, they made only a weak effort to solicit Nathan's and his daughter's input.

Several months later there had been little progress. Nathan remained withdrawn and his weakness and bowel problems were progressing. At that point Nathan was referred to SAF by his primary care physician for outpatient psychiatric treatment and help with coordination of his outpatient care. Regular communication among all those involved, as well as Nathan and his daughter; periodic status reports; and monthly team meetings were instituted. With these changes, Nathan soon began to cooperate with his treatment team, and, as might be expected, his combined systemic medical–psychiatric condition began to stabilize. SAF's function in his coordinating role was quite different from that of a consultant, including the hospital psychosomatic psychiatrist.

This example should help make the case for the advantage of having an MPCP as coordinator for complex cases like Nathan's. Nonetheless, there are still unaddressed issues including the cost and practicality of this method of care delivery. How, for example, can we justify the cost of adding an additional physician to an already costly treatment? The answer is that problematic, co-morbid systemic medical–psychiatric illness, subjected to imprecise diagnosis and treatment, is likely to be more costly on an ongoing basis than if the clinical care is determined through careful diagnostic procedures and is meticulously strategized (Naughton *et al.*, 1994; Vogeli *et al.*, 2007). Tentative support for this claim comes from our pilot study of 52 patients. We will further discuss this study and other issues involving MPCP care and it implementation in Chapter 11.

The medical–psychiatric coordinating physician: clinical role, training models, costs, and future directions

Topics discussed in this book include "truing," clinical judgment, clinical strategy, and the MPCP model of care. All are pertinent to the practice of good clinical medicine. We envision the MPCP as addressing a specific range of clinical needs. Especially targeted is the comprehensive diagnosis and treatment of the high-resource-utilizing, *management intensive, complex* patients that are frequently encountered in the practices of both psychiatrists and PCPs. Of equal importance for the MPCP's role is the development and ongoing coordination of the multidisciplinary treatment teams created for working with these patients. Our motivation for developing this new model for treatment is to provide a more efficient and patient-centered model of care for this highly visible group of patients.

"Complex" as used here and as was defined in Chapter 1, refers to patients (Table 11.1) with co-morbid and overlapping symptomatology, including systemic medical, psychiatric, and psychosocial requirements ("clinical complexity") that necessitate the services of multiple physician specialists as well as allied health professionals ("operational complexity"), the requirement for frequent medical attention, and a tendency to use resources in a redundant and disorganized manner ("management complexity"). The problems for which these patients come to treatment tend to recur and do not resolve with conventional outpatient treatment. Existing medical specializations cannot easily accommodate these patients, in part because of their confounding systemic medical requirements, but also because the psychiatric and psychosocial features in their presentation challenge the capabilities of most primary care physicians. Illustrations of these kinds of cases are provided in the next section of this chapter. There is little diagnostic uniformity to them; instead they tend to cluster according to their extensive management requirements.

The MPCP model of care is the cornerstone of our project. In this chapter the responsibilities of the MPCP will be outlined, and recommended training and experience for that role will be broached. We also explain why we consider the

Table 11.1 Examples of cases appropriate for the MPCP care model

Solid organ transplant (e.g., liver, kidney)
Hepatitis C (HCV) infection, including psychiatric complications of medications used in treatment e.g., interferon, ribavirin
HIV disease
Systemic lupus erythematosus
Diabetes mellitus with co-morbid psychiatric illness such as depression and vascular dementia
CNS illness with psychiatric co-morbidity e.g., multiple sclerosis, Parkinson's disease, Huntington's disease
Traumatic brain injury
Chronic gastrointestinal illness e.g., inflammatory bowel disease and irritable bowel syndrome
Cancer
Chronic pain
Cases with excessive and/or inefficient utilization of medical resources ("the high utilizer")
Psychiatric illnesses interfering with compliance and comprehension of medical treatment requirements
Non-compliance with medical treatment based on psychosocial factors
Substance abuse complicating medical treatment
Somatoform disorders

MPCP to be a distinctive area of medical practice and possibly a future, designated subspecialty of psychiatry or perhaps a subsubspecialty of Psychosomatic Medicine. In its generic, *Coordinating Physician*, variation, this model of care could also become or contribute to a specialization within internal medicine or family medicine.[1]

The skills of the MPCP overlap with those of general psychiatrists, psychiatrists additionally qualified in Psychosomatic Medicine, dually trained physicians in internal medicine/psychiatry and family medicine/psychiatry, and primary care physicians who take an interest in the psychiatric and psychosocial aspects of the care they deliver. However, the functions of an MPCP are specific, and additional training and experience are advisable for embracing this area of practice. As such, one can envision multiple career pathways leading to specialization as an MPCP [Table 11.2].[2]

---

[1] Certainly, within psychiatry the MPCP could qualify as a "subsubspecialty" of psychosomatic medicine. Alternatively, the MPCP model of care could be conceptualized as a subspecialty for those physicians trained in psychiatry and internal medicine or family medicine.

[2] Of the following chapter sections, those that deal with training for the MPCP ("Becoming an MPCP"), its implementation within different treatment settings ("Implementation"), and financial considerations associated with MPCP work (parts of the section on "Affordability") are tangential to the topic of its clinical application and can be skipped over if desired.

Table 11.2 Potential career paths for MPCP subspecialization

Specialization/subspecialization
Psychiatry
Psychiatry plus Psychosomatic Medicine
Combined Family Medicine or Internal Medicine AND Psychiatry, with concurrent or sequential residencies (and with/without Psychosomatic Medicine qualification)
For functioning as a "Coordinating Physician' according to the MPCP model of care delivery: Internal Medicine or Family Medicine with additional training in psychiatry and the management of multi-person and multidisciplinary systems of social organization and patient care

Examples of outpatient cases appropriate for MPCP care

What do the complex cases to which we refer actually look like? You, of course, have read the extensive case descriptions given in previous chapters. MPCP cases are diagnostically heterogeneous and almost always distinguished by their excessive management requirements. The case examples that follow fall at the more "extreme" end of this spectrum of patients. These patients are more personally compromised, more demanding, and more management intensive than many of the cases we have described in previous chapters. However, they are representative of a sizable segment of the complex cases encountered by PCPs.

Below are three vignettes of cases from a primary care physician's practice. Because of their prominent psychiatric and systemic medical needs they could not be managed successfully by that PCP and would likely have benefitted from MPCP care. In the words of the treating PCP: "If the MPCP could coordinate care for these people or arrange team care, it would relieve the burden for the PCP and more importantly might help the patient in a distinctly more constructive manner. I think having the MPCP trained in both (systemic) medicine and psychiatry is essential and far superior to having either a primary care medical or a psychiatric person do the job. As I've said for a long time, with complex cases like these I often have felt like I am practicing psychiatry without a license."

Case 1: Marsha

Marsha was a 55-year-old retired nurse. She easily became agitated and angry, especially when her sense of order and control was violated. Her dissatisfaction and blaming had alienated her family members. When anxious she chewed on her fingers so viciously that she developed osteomyelitis of one of her thumbs, eventually necessitating a partial amputation. She also had multiple other comorbidities including a past CVA (cerebrovascular accident). Her primary care physician had been unsuccessfully exhorting her for years to see a psychiatrist. She had seen one several years previously. The psychiatrist prescribed risperidone, 2 mg twice a day, assuming her behavior reflected a Borderline Personality Disorder (DSM-IV-TR 301.83). Her chewing slowed, but the medication caused tremors and was then discontinued. Over years the primary care physician attempted to enlist several additional medical and surgical specialists, all of whom were dispatched in short order by the patient.

Case 2: Norma

Norma was a 56-year-old, extremely obese woman with diabetes mellitus and related neuropathy, severe arthritis, as well as a life-threatening requirement for CPAP (continuous positive airway pressure). She had severe claustrophobia, could not tolerate any sort of mask over her face, and required a tracheotomy so she wouldn't suffocate in her sleep. In addition to problems getting her to see and cooperate with specialists such as an endocrinologist and rheumatologist, the PCP had been unsuccessful in treating her with psychotropic medications for both anxiety and neuropathic pain. The PCP did her best to constitute a multi-specialty treatment team for the care of this patient, but was repeatedly thwarted by the patient's thoroughgoing lack of compliance.

Case 3: Paul

Paul was a 66-year-old, morbidly obese man with diabetes mellitus, congestive heart failure aggravated by obesity, and sleep apnea. He admitted that he was a compulsive eater and would not follow a diet even though he had severe diabetic retinopathy, neuropathy, and nephropathy. He was hospitalized periodically with pulmonary edema. He refused to wear a CPAP mask because it felt uncomfortable to him. As in the other two examples, none of the PCP's attempts to enlist and coordinate the required specialty care were successful in addressing the patient's complex requirements.

Case 4: Stanley (continued)

Too far removed from the norm? Return to Stanley from Chapter 1. Recall his claim that he was in excruciating pain and that no previous surgery had helped him.

Stanley, as you may remember, was a 62-year-old veteran of three spinal surgeries and multiple psychotherapies. He had been referred to SAF for assessment and treatment of his psychiatric and neurological problems. He initially received excellent care, but progressively his physicians became exasperated by his complaints and never-ending dissatisfaction, visit by visit losing interest in going the extra mile to treat him. It became clear that simply to manage Stanley's inexorable discontent, centering on his complaints about intolerable pain, his physicians had turned to analgesics, mainly opioids, and increasingly higher doses of barbiturates and benzodiazepines. In their words, "what other choice was

Table 11.3 The MPCP's proposed job description

Planning and strategizing duties	Microscopic responsibilities involving treatment team management	Macroscopic responsibilities involving treatment team management	Outcome assessment	Direct patient treatment
Assembles clinical team	Maintains team cohesion through discussions with individual team members and team meetings	Assumes the leadership role in multiple specialist treatment teams	Collaboratively develops outcome measures and is responsible for following and revising these throughout treatment	Generally provides some aspects of direct treatment e.g., psychotherapy, prescribing psychotropic medications
Coordination, formulation, and negotiation of overall treatment plan	Initiates and guides treatment plan implementation and revisions	Coordination of medical and surgical workups, and resulting treatments	Ongoing assessment of the validity of the treatment plan	Serves as liaison to patient and to family of patient, as permitted by patient
Ongoing strategizing and prioritizing of team-originated and individual-team-member-initiated treatment interventions	Responsible for communicating clinical data, and finding and sharing new case-related technical information with team members	Management of the patient's entire, case-related, "psychosocial-medical" system	Seeks regular reports from team members and agencies	MPCP views his or her job as in some manner "treating" the patient's entire, case-related, "biopsychosocial-medical" system
Control of treatment quality; insuring that treatments used are appropriate and as possible evidence-based			Shares determinations of treatment progress with team members and patient	

there?" What had been a case for a neurosurgeon became one for a psychiatrist working hand in hand with a PCP. Continued care then required a decisive change in strategy including reassembling Stanley's physicians into a treatment team. At that point SAF became the MPCP, organizing and directing this team and providing the psychiatric care as well.

Case 5: Organ transplantation patient

Organ transplantation is another, frequently encountered complex medical–psychiatric situation – one for which the MPCP role is ideally suited. The following multi-dimensional case serves as an example of such a situation, with the eventual development of an MPCP-like arrangement to provide the patient's care.

The patient, a 50-year-old, married, high-functioning woman, developed a silent dependence on alcohol over the course of many years. She had spent years hiding her dependence from others, including her attentive husband and family. The only outward manifestations that she might have a problem were escalating gastrointestinal and musculoskeletal complaints. These issues were treated symptomatically. Her addiction was only made public after she twice vomited blood.

The patient's drinking continued, however. Over time cirrhosis was diagnosed, the patient's liver disease progressing to the point where she required a liver transplant. Multiple physicians were recruited to consult on the case as she awaited liver transplantation. During this period she temporarily stopped using alcohol and attended Alcoholics Anonymous (AA). Although the anticipation of the procedure was arduous for the patient, the transplant was successful and her hospital course uneventful except for an episode of delirium that was associated with delusions about the hospital staff. This episode resolved after treatment with olanzapine.

The patient did well after discharge and was compliant with medical treatment. Follow-up involved treatment with post-transplant anti-rejection medications, combined psychopharmacological treatment, and psychotherapy, as well as active participation in AA. Critical to her ultimate success was close, MPCP-like cooperative management by her primary care physician and psychiatrist.

In addition to the commingling of psychiatric and systemic medical illness, the clinical picture in this case was complicated by co-morbid substance dependence eventuating in liver disease. Treatment of the "whole patient," in a manner consistent with the MPCP model, was ultimately necessary for the patient to attain comprehensive clinical improvement and sustain a successful adjustment to the rigors of post-transplant management. In retrospect, however, the organization and treatment of the case, both pre- and post-transplant, would likely have been more efficiently and economically managed by the involvement of an actual MPCP.

The MPCP's job description

It seems reasonable to compare MPCP responsibilities to that of a psychosomatic psychiatrist (Leentjens et al., 2011), since both work at the interface of psychiatry

Table 11.4 Summary of the MPCP's point-by-point role in patient care

The MPCP:
(1) Assesses the complexity of the clinical situation, noting and prioritizing its components. In addition, the MPCP continually integrates input from team members, while searching for new, clinically relevant, information.
(2) Selects the clinical aspects to focus on at each point as the case progresses.
(3) Coordinates all team members, integrating and interpreting each one's contribution.
(4) Monitors clinical progress, continually communicating and discussing new findings with team members and integrating these into the treatment plan.
(5) Applies "truing" measures, including those associated with the "conjunctive method" (Chapter 9), to guide the work of team members individually and the team collectively.
(6) Fills a different role from that of a typical medical team coordinator or primary care physician by taking both a microscopic and macroscopic view of the patient's and team's management requirements. In addition, the MPCP also brings to bear the experience and judgment of a physician so relevant in clinically and operationally complex, management-intensive, cases.
(7) Delivers some or all of the psychiatric care required by the patient.

and systemic medicine and are inclined to deal with "clinically complex" patients. While an MPCP's duties (Table 11.3) in some ways overlap those of a psychiatrist with training in psychosomatic medicine, there are important distinctions. These include the MPCP's point-by-point involvement in *ongoing* treatments (Table 11.4). Added, is the leadership role with the multiple specialist teams frequently associated with these cases, comprehensive and sustained case management that includes addressing prominent psychosocial issues, and active coordination of workups, whether systemic medical, surgical, or a combination thereof.

In effect, then, the MPCP has the specific charge of organizing and administering the patient's problematic social, psychiatric, and systemic medical requirements. An MPCP may also provide an important part in the patient's direct treatment, and/or, within that role, prescribe psychotropic medication, carry out psychotherapy, or aspects of the patient's systemic medical care. If the MPCP is also qualified in internal medicine or family medicine, he or she could also function as PCP for the case. Repeating a point made several times earlier, MPCP patient care has the greatest practical utility for ongoing work with cases with psychiatric co-morbidity and complex management requirements necessitating the involvement of several interacting professionals. It stands to reason, then, that in these cases, it is desirable and often mandatory that the MPCP be a psychiatrist.

Skills required of an MPCP

Given the comprehensive nature of the MPCP's activities, the training and exposure requirements for this work are specific (Tables 11.5 and Tables 11.6).

Table 11.5 Background and skills pertinent to MPCP subspecialization

---

Skill with formulating clinical strategy, as well as creating and prioritizing interventions in complex cases; required is the capacity to use medical, psychodynamic, behavioral, social systems, and management principles to this end

Working knowledge of developmental theory and its application to understanding patients and families, as well as their interactions between themselves and with society

Understanding of and experience working with families

Understanding and working with treatment-associated professional groups, including treatment teams

Skill with facilitating collaboration between professionals and in conflict resolution

Familiarity with the work of medical specialists who are likely to constitute treatment teams

Understanding "Level 1" and "Level 2" truing measures

Acquaintance with case-relevant cultural issues and their impact on treatment

Working knowledge of care delivery systems and financial matters involved in delivery of care

Understanding and applying methods for determining and following treatment progress, creating and using outcome measures

Familiarity with diagnosis and treatment at the interface of systemic medicine and psychiatry, including subjects particular to psychosomatic medicine such as decisional capacity determinations

---

While many of the basic skills will have been learned in residency, in particular a general psychiatry, combined general psychiatry and internal medicine or family medicine residency, or in a psychosomatic medicine fellowship, others are specific to the MPCP role. Skills required to function as a non-psychiatric "Coordinating Physician" could, in addition to post-graduate training in internal medicine, family medicine, or pediatrics, be gained in seminars and continuing education courses or a fellowship devoted to teaching the MPCP model.

Familiarity with individual, family, and group psychology, as well as the structure and workings of professional hierarchies, is essential for engaging in MPCP work. For the role of treatment-team coordinator, basic instruction in group dynamics and its potential complications, together with supervised hands-on experience with groups and families, is essential. Added, is clinical exposure to families associated with complex cases and highlighting the effect family members have on one another, as well as the impact of the patient and his or her illnesses on family members.

From a macroscopic perspective, the MPCP has the pivotal management role in the patient's entire, case-related systemic medical and psychosocial system. Included here are the multiple physician specialists, consultants, and allied health professionals who are involved in the case, as well as, frequently, the patient's family and representatives from his or her social and cultural world. Here, the MPCP is operating in a high-level coordinating capacity, insuring that the multiple constituencies of the treatment system provide input and interact productively with one another. To assure his or her effectiveness as treatment coordinator, the MPCP should also be familiar with each team member's clinical specialty.

Table 11.6 Proposed training topics for the MPCP role

Orientation to the MPCP method of patient care and care delivery: its structure, indications, and supporting theories

The place of the MPCP method in outpatient systems and hospitals, and in the fee-for-service system

Healthcare delivery systems: history, models, and economics; their relevance for the MPCP model of care

The MPCP's role in appraising, working-up, and strategizing complex cases

The treatment team: its creation and management; the coordinating role of the MPCP

The psychology and management of the family in the treatment of complex cases

The *ongoing* MPCP management of complex cases, including selecting, ordering, and prioritizing clinical interventions

Principles of optimizing treatment using "truing" measures as applied by (1) individual physician team members and (2) the MPCP at the level of team coordination

Practical issues in the interfacing of an MPCP-coordinated team with case-related organizations, including agencies, schools, hospitals

Case conferences

Relevant technical topics in systemic medicine and psychiatry:

· Review of systemic illnesses with significant psychiatric co-morbidity

· Management of psychotropic medications in medically ill patients

· Drug–drug interactions

· Psychotherapy models and their application to systemically ill patients

Understanding and working with the psychology and sociology of interconnected personal, social, and medical systems

Collaboration between medical professionals: how it succeeds or fails

Treatment modalities in psychiatry and psychology that are pertinent to the work of an MPCP

Cultural issues and biostatistics

As strategist-coordinator for the treatment team, the MPCP determines and uses outcome measures to track and provide direction for the clinical work. He or she relies on these for developing, following, and modifying the patient's treatment plan. Monitoring treatment requires familiarity with truing measures for gauging and optimizing clinical progress, and necessitates continuous screening of the medical literature for information pertinent to the case. Taken together, all these aspects of the MPCP's work provide the data for one of the MPCP's most important activities, the prioritizing and strategizing of team decisions and actions.

The MPCP's place as team coordinator and in managing conflict within the treatment team

From within the team, the MPCP's coordinating function might come into play as follows. This is an example of the ever-present "social" component of the biopsychosocial perspective that an MPCP needs to keep in mind. (1) Dr. A., the primary physician in the case, comes in at 8:00 a.m., writes orders, and communicates her clinical opinion to the patient and nursing staff. Dr. B., from a different service and senior to Dr. A., comes in at 10:00 and modifies Dr. A.'s orders, leaving the patient bewildered and the nursing staff in a quandary about which orders to follow. (2) Dr. A., however, has already communicated her opinion to the patient's family, and Dr. B.'s conflicting position leaves the family perplexed and even worried about the nature and quality of care their family member is receiving. (3) Dr. A. and Dr. B. have done their best to talk with each other but, because of their busy schedules, have to play telephone tag. They are unable to make contact until several hours after this order-writing scenario is over.

With this example in hand, return to the skills and flexibility required for the MPCP to effectively create and manage treatment teams. Clearly, as illustrated in the example above, the MPCP, while in the role of coordinator, has to account for the impact of each member on team functioning. Expertise in conflict resolution is required for the MPCP to negotiate successfully between team members as inevitable differences between them arise. Also, along with his or her other roles, the MPCP needs to be in regular communication with the patient and often the patient's family. The objective of this activity is for the MPCP to remain current about the patient's and family's needs and attitudes, as well as to keep in close touch with important clinical developments. In this role the MPCP is a personal resource for the patient and family (Table 11.5).

Becoming an MPCP

Here we add some thoughts about training for the MPCP. However, since training is not the focus of this book, we leave the details to future publications devoted to that subject.

We picture the bulk of MPCP training as taking place within psychiatry residency and fellowship education, as well as post-specialty training programs offering continuing education credit. Ideally, as the MPCP model takes hold, this training could be encompassed within a separate MPCP-themed fellowship. Since the MPCP is a new care delivery model with conceptual overlap and clinical "fit" with psychosomatic medicine as well as with combined internal medicine/psychiatry and family medicine/psychiatry, a logical first place for implementing this training would be within existing psychosomatic fellowships and internal medicine/psychiatry and family medicine/psychiatry training programs.[3] For the fully trained physician who wishes to pursue

---

[3] Given that these programs already have significant training needs, it would perhaps be unrealistic at this point to expect that such training programs could begin by devoting more than 10% of clinical time for a single academic year to this model. For such experiences, trainees could benefit from a supervised experience where they take on the MPCP role for the complex patients we have described throughout this book. A series of directed readings and seminars on the relevant literature would accompany the clinical work (Table 11.6).

competence in the MPCP model, a series of continuing medical education courses and supervised clinical experiences, or even a fellowship, could be offered.[4]

Table 11.6 presents elements of a proposed curriculum for residency or fellowship-based training. Of course, there are many ways this instruction can be organized, providing that it enlarges on the candidate's previous education in psychiatry and systemic medicine, and is focused on the application of psychiatric–systemic medical care for complex cases. Added to the course work and practical instruction identified in Table 11.6 could be training in organizational dynamics and technology, such as that incorporated into Masters of Public Health (MPH), Masters of Public Administration (MPA), or Masters of Business Administration (MBA) programs. Relevant topics from those programs could be included in the core MPCP training program, offered as electives, or be available as ongoing training.

Models for MPCP training are under development and are only proposed at this point. For example, we can envision a full academic year longitudinal elective that occupies 10% of the time of a Psychosomatic Medicine (PM) fellowship or the fifth year of a Combined Internal Medicine and Psychiatry (Med/Psych) or combined family medicine and psychiatry (FM/Psych) residency. A reasonable time requirement for such training might be 4 hours a week for 50 weeks, or a total of 200 hours for the academic year. Components of a model curriculum are outlined in Table 11.6 and could be accompanied by a half-day, weekly complex-case clinic.

The MPCP's training and experience could also extend to several subsidiary areas not included in Table 11. 6. Added might be the understanding and management of cost containment issues, issues associated with fostering ongoing credibility with members of a treatment team, mediating disagreements between team members, and formally tracking patient progress.[5]

What is a medical specialization?

Specializations aren't made in heaven. They arise because they are needed (Cassel & Ruben, 2011). And, indeed, that appears to be the situation with

---

[4] For example, if this training were 50 hours in duration, included might be a 3-hour introduction to the MPCP model; and a series of 6-hour workshops on pertinent topics such as: complex patients and their care, medical–psychiatric co-morbidity and management, and team management. All offerings could be designed to mirror the proposed model for training within institutional programs.

[5] As we envision it, MPCP may be an ideal job choice for physicians interested in the outpatient application of psychosomatic medicine, or those with combined training and an interest in the psychosocial issues that invariably permeate complex treatments. To date, graduates of these combined programs have tended to gravitate toward positions with primary care, internal medicine/family practice, or psychiatry, with some taking positions on the limited number of medical–psychiatry services in hospitals. Hence, the MPCP is a career that is likely to be ready-made for these dual-trained physicians: a career where their combined skills could be practiced optimally.

Table 11.7 Examples of specialties and subspecialties of internal medicine and psychiatry

Internal medicine	Psychiatry
Adolescent Medicine	Addiction Psychiatry
Advanced Heart Failure and Transplant	Child and Adolescent Psychiatry
Cardiology	Forensic Psychiatry
Allergy and Immunology	Geriatric Psychiatry
Cardiovascular Disease	Pain Medicine
Clinical Cardiac Electrophysiology	Psychosomatic Medicine
Critical Care Medicine	Specializations within Psychosomatic
Endocrinology, Diabetes, and Metabolism	Medicine:
Gastroenterology	Psycho-Oncology
Geriatric Medicine	Transplant Psychiatry
Hematology	HIV Psychiatry
Hospice and Palliative Medicine	
Infectious Disease	
Interventional Cardiology	
Medical Oncology	
Nephrology	
Pulmonary Disease	
Rheumatology	
Sleep Medicine	
Sports Medicine	
Transplant Hepatology	

the MPCP. We envision the MPCP as having a specific role in the organization and ongoing treatment of complex cases, such as those represented in Table 11.7. We have already mentioned three seemingly similar specializations with systemic medical–psychiatric emphasis: psychosomatic medicine (PM), combined internal medicine and psychiatry (Med/Psych), and combined family medicine and psychiatry (FM/Psych). All three deal with complex patients with co-morbid medical–psychiatric illness. None of these, however, specifically focuses on physician coordination of the multiple specialists required in the treatment of complex cases, and the involved physician's responsibility for tracking and optimizing long-term outcome.

Returning to recognized subspecialties. There are a plethora of these in internal medicine and psychiatry. Table 11.7 calls attention to their diversity. Physicians practicing in each listed subspecialty have completed a residency in general psychiatry or internal medicine prior to pursuing further qualification in the subspecialty. Training in the mentioned "combination" specializations, internal medicine/psychiatry and family medicine/psychiatry requires a total of 5 years of split residency training; for example, 2½ years in internal medicine and 2½ years in psychiatry.

Outpatient psychosomatic medicine: an opportunity for MPCP practice?

Psychosomatic medicine (PM) (Gitlin, 2004; Leentjens *et al.*, 2011) should serve as an example for us, as we consider whether the MPCP may ultimately qualify as a subspecialty of psychiatry or "sub-subspecialty" of a psychiatric subspecialty such as psychosomatic medicine. Psychosomatic medicine is a subspecialty of psychiatry concerned with the diagnosis and treatment of psychiatric disorders in medically ill patients. Psychosomatic medicine psychiatrists have traditionally provided consultation for patients with medical or surgical illness with co-morbid psychiatric manifestations (see Table 11.8). These patients also may have psychiatric disorders that are the direct consequence of systemic medical conditions and/or somatoform disorders.

Psychiatrists specializing in psychosomatic medicine serve on consultation-liaison services in general medical hospitals, attend on medical–psychiatry inpatient units, and have been integrated into the "collaborative care" programs offered in primary care and other outpatient settings. However, in these situations PM psychiatrists remain consultants to primary treating physicians. Expanding on the PM psychiatrist's traditional role is the increasing emphasis on outpatient care in PM training programs and practice (Bourgeois *et al.*, 2003, 2005; Rundell *et al.*, 2008), a clinical role with which the MPCP's focus on ongoing, closely monitored treatment should fit nicely.

The spectrum of patients that fall within the PM psychiatrist's repertoire, then, are generally also appropriate for MPCP care. However, as noted, the responsibilities of the MPCP are in important ways different from those of PM psychiatrists. Emphasized in the MPCP's work are the ongoing management of complex cases involving systemic medical and psychiatric co-morbid illness, treatment team formation and coordination, and responsibility for optimization of results. The contrast between the MPCP's focus on case management and outcome with the PM psychiatrist's typically more focal role as consultant to other physicians highlights the difference between the two.

It seems worth noting that the work of the PM psychiatrist and MPCP both benefit from an understanding of the interaction of social, cultural, psychological, and behavioral factors with bodily processes and their malfunctions. However, while the issues identified here are of importance for the consultation function of a PM psychiatrist, the MPCP has the expanded charge of working with them in depth and over time. Added, is the MPCP's responsibility for providing connection between members of the treatment team, as well as between the treatment team, the patient, and frequently his or her family.

In summary, specific to the MPCP are the ongoing evaluation, organization, and coordination of all facets of the patient's systemic medical–psychosocial system. The MPCP incrementally addresses malfunctions of that system and does this work in collaboration with other specialists who are organized and

Table 11.8 Typical responsibilities of a Psychosomatic Medicine psychiatrist: an example of a Psychiatric subspecialization

Basic concept	Responsibilities	Examples of categories of patients
Subspecialization in the diagnosis and treatment of psychiatric disorders and symptoms in complex, medically ill patients	Consultation for patients with acute or chronic medical, neurological, obstetrical, or surgical illness, and with co-morbid psychiatric illness	Specific systemic disease states: HIV/AIDS disease, HCV infection (hepatitis C), organ transplantation, heart disease, renal failure, cancer, neurodegenerative illness, stroke, traumatic brain injury, chronic obstructive pulmonary disease (COPD), complications of pregnancy, rheumatologic diseases, endocrinological illness
	Liaison services that link the medical team and the patient. These services are found in the general medical hospital, in association with medical–psychiatry inpatient units, and provide integration with collaborative care programs in primary care and other outpatient settings	Patients with challenges adapting to their illnesses: patients with chronic systemic disease with its associated psychosocial complications patients who over-utilize healthcare
		Ambiguous "psychosomatic presentations" of illness: somatization disorder, hypochondriasis, conversion disorder

managed by the MPCP as a treatment team. Stated succinctly, the MPCP is the *physician from the group of medical practitioners that treat complex patients who takes on the most pointedly integrative medical and psychosocial charge.*

Affordability

We anticipate concern being raised that having a physician as treatment coordinator unreasonably increases costs, at least early in treatment. However, when considering this issue note that treatment of complex patients who make excessive, chaotic, or repetitive use of specialists, and where the role of psychiatric co-morbidity is a key clinical feature, is already associated with significantly increased costs as well as inferior functional outcomes (Katon *et al.*, 1990; Kathol & Gatteau, 2007; Vogeli *et al.*, 2007; Atlas, 2009; Gawande *et al.*, 2009; Leff *et al.*, 2009).

In contrast, MPCP leadership is by design associated with the efficient use and coordination of specialists, judicious utilization of resources, and the earlier identification and more timely management of clinical problems. When these features are considered together with the MPCP's ability to co-manage psychiatric co-morbidity, we are persuaded that the clinical advantages of the MPCP model for treatment of complex cases can reliably translate into cost offset. In our opinion the economy of this approach should prevail in spite of the increased "overhead" that is especially apparent towards the beginning of treatment.

Other, less-tangible contributions to cost savings from an MPCP approach derive from improved treatment compliance that often results from close attention by the MPCP to patients' medical and related psychosocial needs and the alliance that often forms between the two as a result. Also, the MPCP is continuously available to provide information to help patients understand and manage their needs, as well as to identify preventative measures to forestall progression of illness.

At this point, our confidence in the future advantages of the MPCP model comes from the more than 50 outpatient cases completed using this model, each treated for over 18 months by two of the authors of this book (Table 11.9). Case retention was impressive for our pilot group (Table 11.9). Judging from repeated, anonymous patient surveys taken during and following their treatments, these patients generally experienced high levels of satisfaction, reliable symptom resolution, improvement in the quality of their lives, and a sense that their medical and psychiatric needs had been understood and taken seriously.

Our pilot project consisted of 52 outpatient cases treated by one of the authors of this paper (SAF) and another seasoned clinician, each for at least 18 months. Comprehensive chart review indicated sustained improvement in at least two clinical dimensions in 44 patients following adoption of the MPCP model. Outcome criteria included reduced utilization of resources including emergency room visits and hospitalizations, increased treatment adherence, decrease in systemic medical or psychiatric symptoms (by rating scales), and improved quality of life (by rating scales). Subjects were selected from a pool of office-based patients according to the following criteria: at least two other physicians had been previously involved in their care, at least one other ongoing treatment had been attempted, and the patient required frequent extra visits, and phone calls or emails for their support.

Also, two of us (SAF and PE) have used variations of the MPCP method in our practices for over 20 years. We have also conducted two additional clinical projects dedicated to the creation of a collaborative treatment model, as the MPCP model was being developed. Each project involved a sizable sample of patients, treated over a several-year period. PE and SAF worked in partnership as

Table 11.9 Summary of 52 treated cases

Patient number	Age	Gender	Systemic medical diagnoses	Psychiatric diagnoses (secondary diagnoses in parentheses)	Number of consultants	Number of involved family members	Outcome (see below for legend)
1	67	F	MUPS, ND	A	6	5	RU TA
2	16	M	GI	DID	3	2	TA Sx Q
3	50	F	MUPS	SD, A	4	3	RU TA Sx
4	16	F		D-S (SD)	6	2	TA Sx
5	49	M		A, Som	3	0	RU TA Sx Q
6	24	F	MUPS, FM	SD	3	2	RU TA
7	42	M		D-S, BPD	2	2	RU TA Sx Q
8	41	M		BAD, ADD	3	2	RU TA Sx Q
9	48	F	MUPS	D, r/o BAD	2	3	RU TA
10	43	M		BAD	2	2	RU TA Sx Q
11	42	F	MUPS	D	1	2	Sx Q
12	30	M	MUPS	Asp	3	3	RU Sx Q
13	24	M		D-S	1	2	Sx Q
14	51	M		BAD	1	0	Sx Q
15	50	F	MUPS, Kid	BAD, D-S, r/o Schiz	3	4	RU Sx
16	18	F		ED	2	2	TA Sx Q
17	61	F	MUPS, Spinal, Ophth, FM	Schiz, D-S	2	1	TA Sx
18	30	M	Spinal, Ortho	CD, Schiz (SD)	4	2	RU TA Sx Q
19	18	M		ADD with CD, OCD, SD	3	2	RU TA Sx Q
20	49	M	BT, EL	D	4	2	TA Sx
21	60	M	MD, EL	A (SD)	4	1	RU TA Q
22	71	M	PV, EL	A, D	4	4	RU TA Q
23	68	F	Scl	D	4	2	TA Sx Q
24	76	M	Park	D	3	1	RU TA Sx Q
25	58	F	FM, r/o MS	Som, BPD	4	2	RU TA
26	59	F	MUPS, CFS	D, r/o Schiz	4	2	RU TA Sx Q

Table 11.9 (cont.)

Patient number	Age	Gender	Systemic medical diagnoses	Psychiatric diagnoses (secondary diagnoses in parentheses)	Number of consultants	Number of involved family members	Outcome (see below for legend)
27	30	M	MUPS	SD	4	4	RU TA Sx Q
28	18	F		A, ADD (SD)	3	3	RU TA Q
29	17	F		BAD, ED	3	3	Sx Q
30	19	F	MUPS	BAD (SD)	3	3	Sx Q
31	15	F		CD (SD)	2	5	TA Sx
32	26	M	Ortho	SD, r/o BPD	4	3	TA Sx Q
33	72	F	MUPS	A, BPD (SD)	3	4	RU TA Sx Q
34	12	F	GI	ED	4	1	TA Sx
35	26	M		D (SD)	2	3	TA Sx Q
36	15	M		CD (SD, ADD)	3	4	TA Sx
37	65	F	CFS	PTSD	4	0	Sx Q
38	30	M	MUPS	CD	3	3	RU TA
39	19	M	MUPS	Schiz (CD, SD)	4+	2	RU TA
40	50	M	MUPS	A, OCD	3	0	TA Sx
41	65	M	MUPS	A	2	2	RU Sx
42	66	F		PTSD, A	3	0	RU Sx Q
43	67	M	MUPS	PTSD	2	1	RU Sx Q
44	21	F		PTSD, BPD (SD)	3	1	TA Sx
45	48	F	MUPS	D, r/o BAD, Som	2	3	N/C
46	60	F	MUPS	D, BPD	3	1	N/C
47	51	F	MUPS, CFS	D	4	1	N/C
48	45	M		CD, BPD	2	1	N/C
49	41	F	MUPS	CD, D	1	0	N/C
50	25	F		ED (SD)	4	2	N/C
51	14	M		ADD	1	2	N/C
52	62	M	Spinal, MUPS	D, BPD (SD)	6	0	N/C

Abbreviations – systemic medical

r/o = rule out
BT = brain tumor
CFS = chronic fatigue syndrome
EL = end of life
FM = fibromyalgia
GI = gastrointestinal
Kid = renal disease
MD = myelodysplasia
MS = multiple sclerosis
MUPS = multiple unexplained physical symptoms
ND = neurodegenerative disease, with dementia
Ophth = ophthalmological disorder
Ortho = orthopedic
Park = Parkinson's disease
PV = polycythemia vera
Scl = scleroderma
Spinal = spinal nerve, spinal cord injury

Abbreviations – psychiatric

A = anxiety disorder
ADD = attention deficit disorder
Asp = Asperger's syndrome
BPD = borderline personality disorder
BAD = bipolar affective disorder
CD = conduct disorder
D = depressive disorder
DID = dissociative identity disorder
D-S = depressive disorder plus suicidality
ED = eating disorder
OCD = obsessive compulsive disorder
PTSD = posttraumatic stress disorder
Schiz = schizophrenia and other psychotic disorders
SD = substance dependence
Som = somatization disorder

Table 11.9 (*cont.*)

Abbreviations – outcomes

N/C = no change

Q = distinct improvement in quality of life, by patient report

RU (reduced utilization) = one-third fewer calls and visits to PCP/MPCP judged at successive 6-month intervals. No increase in number of unessential specialists over course of treatment. Half as many Emergency Department visits and decreased hospitalizations, compared with the previous two years

Sx = distinct symptomatic improvement, using self assessment rating scales e.g., Hamilton or Beck anxiety and depression scales

TA = improved treatment adherence, by physician report

Summary of outcome

Comprehensive chart review during and following treatment indicated sustained improvement in at least two clinical dimensions in 44 of the 52 patients following adoption of the MPCP model. Outcome criteria included changes in utilization of resources including emergency room visits and hospitalizations, treatment adherence, change in systemic medical or psychiatric symptoms (by rating scales), and shifts in reported quality of life (by rating scales). Patients were selected from a pool of office-based patients according to the following criteria: at least two other professionals had been involved in their care; at least one other treatment had been attempted previously; the patient required frequent extra visits, phone calls, or emails for their support.

they conducted these clinical studies, and SAF has written about them in his other books (Frankel, S., 1995, 2000, 2007, 2008).

Our data from this pilot project supports the view that among the most appropriate cases for MPCP management are those involving complex and chronic illnesses. All the cases studied in our pilot project had significant psychiatric co-morbidity, and all of the patients required the attention of several physicians for their care. In our sample, in addition to the MPCP, there was an average of approximately three physicians involved with each treatment team. Judging from our study, no particular set of medical or psychiatric diagnoses stood out as typical for this cohort of patients. It was the *clinical complexity* of these patients, together with the extensive management they required, that was most characteristic of these cases.

Implementation

We have presented a new model for care delivery for clinically and operationally complex cases, and the outlines of a program for training those who deliver that care. How can this model be put into practice within the current healthcare system?

Claims of efficiency and cost savings are one thing, but how truly effective and patient centered are our healthcare systems, especially when dealing with management-intensive cases? What is sacrificed in the name of economy or resource containment? Altogether, the complications and contradictions in healthcare delivery as it currently exists are daunting. For example, rules erected to contain costs and restrict over-utilization often have the unfortunate effect of limiting patient access to needed healthcare.

As noted above, complex patients tend to require multiple specialists – physicians and otherwise. However, when several physicians and allied healthcare professionals are involved in a case, follow-through is often spotty, with com-munication erratic (Kathol *et al.*, 2010a; Rundell, 2010). The Patient-Centered Medical Home (PCMH) model (Backer, 2007, 2009; Bodenheimer, 2007; Rogers, 2008; Nutting *et al.*, 2009; Stange *et al.*, 2010; Katon & Unützer, 2011), empha-sizing coordinated care, and incorporating a viable electronic record and com-munication system, is an attractive potential antidote to these problems. However, PCMHs are currently just being implemented and evaluated for economy and efficacy. We wonder, how can the issue of cost and resource limitation be dealt with in these situations without making compromises similar to those that have come to characterize other care delivery systems?

Considering these limitations, it seems logical and constructive to recommend implementation of the MPCP model of care for inclusion within existing health-care organizations. In addition to PCMHs, academic medical centers, "closed" healthcare systems such as the Veterans Administration and Department of Defense, or systems that support multispecialty and interdisciplinary care without added financial barriers such as Kaiser Permanente, the Mayo Clinic, and the Cleveland Clinic might be ideal locations for implementing the model.

In evaluating this proposal, recall that in managed care settings the use of non-physician health professionals is generally considered cost-effective and, therefore, that these healthcare practitioners tend to be chosen as case managers (Plsek & Greenhalgh 2001; Latour *et al.*, 2007a, 2007b; Kathol *et al.*, 2010a). However, our experience with the group of management-intensive, complex patients we have identified in this and previous chapters challenges this preference. According to our experience in treating this category of patient, having a physician, and in particular a psychiatrist, in the leadership role in their treatments may well have significant long-term advantages in both cost savings and quality of care.

The future of the MPCP model

In concluding this book we shift to the subject of research for evaluating the efficacy of the MPCP model for the treatment of clinically and operationally complex cases. Definitive studies of this population are likely to be challenging. A short list of considerations as these studies are being designed includes the multiple symptoms with which these patients present, their coexisting diseases, the nature of their personal lives, and the type of care they receive. Also, study subjects should be followed for a reasonable period of time and the expected progression of each of their diseases taken into consideration. Of relevance, also, in selecting research methodology for these studies is whether and how to follow the patients' subjective responses to their illnesses, expressed, for example, as satisfaction with their care, and which objective criteria, such as symptom resolution and frequency of emergency room visits or hospitalizations, to monitor.

We are in the early stages in the development and implementation of the MPCP model, having completed our pilot study. We are encouraged both by our findings and the clinical advantages we and our colleagues have experienced when using this method. We are designing and implementing studies where subjects treated using the MPCP method are compared with those treated with other modalities. Outcome criteria are likely to include such factors as the cost of treatment, symptom resolution, improved life adjustment, and control over the utilization of resources.

As these studies are being launched, we offer the MPCP model of patient care as a logical interim response to the requirement for efficient, effective, and cost-contained treatment for the most challenging group of complex, management-intensive cases. Its comprehensiveness and constructive impact on the quality of care delivered should be welcomed as an antidote to the shortcomings of the more commonly employed, less integrated, and, in many situations, less sophisticated approaches to treating these patients.

References

Abelson, R. P. (1985). A variance explanation paradox: when a little is a lot. *Psychol. Bull.*, **97**, 129–133.

American College of Physicians. (2006). The Advanced Medical Home: A Patient-Centered, Physician-Guided Model of Health Care. (Position paper.) Philadelphia, PA: American College of Physicians.

American Diabetes Association. (2012). Standards of medical care in diabetes – 2012. (Position paper.) *Diabetes Care*, **35 Suppl. 1**, S11–S63. doi: 10.2337/dc12-s011

American Psychiatric Association. (2000). Diagnostic and Statistical Manual of Mental Disorders (DSM-IV-TR), 4th edn., rev. Washington DC: American Psychiatric Association.

Arkes, H. R. (1981). Impediments to accurate clinical judgment and possible ways to minimize their impact. *J. Consult. Clin. Psychol.*, **49**, 323–330.

Aron, L. (1991). The patient's experience of the analyst's subjectivity. *Psychoanal. Dialog.*, **1**(1), 29–51.

Aron, L. (1992). Interpretation as expression of the analyst's subjectivity. *Psychoanal. Dialog.*, **2**(4), 475–508.

Aron, L. (1996). A Meeting of the Minds: Mutuality in Psychoanalysis. Hillsdale, NJ: Analytic Press.

Atlas, S. J. (2009). Patient-physician connectedness and quality of primary care. *Ann. Intern. Med.*, **150**, 325–335.

Backer, L. A. (2007). The medical home: an idea whose time has come … again. *Fam. Pract. Manag.*, **14**, 38–41.

Backer, L. A. (2009). Building the case for the patient-centered medical home. *Fam. Pract. Manag.*, **16**(1), 14–18.

Barber, J. P., Connolly, M. B., Crits-Christoph, P., Gladis, L., & Siqueland, L. (2000). Alliance predicts patients' outcome beyond in-treatment change in symptoms. *J. Consult. Clin. Psychol.*, **68**, 1027–1032.

Beck, A. T., Steer, R. A., & Brown, G. K. (1996). Beck Depression Inventory-II (BDI-II). San Antonio, TX: Psychological Corp.

Beebe, B. & Lachmann, F. M. (2002). Infant Research and Adult Treatment: Co-constructing Interactions. Hillsdale, NJ: Analytic Press.

Ben-Porath, Y. S. & Tellegen, A. (2008). Minnesota Multiphasic Personality Inventory-2 Restructured Form: Manual for Administration, Scoring, and Interpretation. Minneapolis, MN: University of Minnesota Press.

Berwick, D. (2008). The epitaph of profession. *Br. J. Gen. Pract.*, **59**, 128–131.

Beutler, L. (2009). Making science matter in clinical practice: redefining psychotherapy. *Clin. Psychol. Sci. Prac.*, **16**(3), 302–317.

Bickman, L. (2008). A measurement feedback system (MFS) is necessary to improve mental health outcomes. *J. Am. Acad. Child Adolesc. Psychiatry*, **47**, 10.

Bodenheimer, T. (2007). Building Teams in Primary Care: Fifteen Case Studies. Oakland, CA: California HealthCare Foundation.

Bogan, C. E. & English, M. J. (1994). Benchmarking for Best Practices: Winning through Innovative Adaptation. New York: McGraw Hill.

Bohmer, R. & Lee, T. (2009). The shifting mission of health care delivery organizations. *N. Engl. J. Med.*, **361**(6), 551–553.

Borum, R., Otto, R., & Golding, S. (1993). Improving clinical judgment and decision making in forensic evaluation. *J. Psychiatry Law*, **21**, 35–76.

Bourgeois, J. A., Hilty, D. M., Klein, S. C., *et al.* (2003). Expansion of the consultation-liaison psychiatry paradigm at a university medical center: integration of diversified clinical and funding models. *Gen. Hosp. Psychiatry*, **25**, 262–268.

Bourgeois, J. A., Hilty, D. M., Servis, M. E., & Hales, R. E. (2005). Consultation-liaison psychiatry advantages for healthcare systems: review article. *Dis. Manag. Health Out.*, **13**(2), 93–106.

Bourgeois, J. A., Kahn, D., Philbrick, K. L., & Bostwick, J. M. (2008). Casebook of Psychosomatic Medicine. Washington DC: American Psychiatric Publishing Inc.

Campbell, D. T. & Fiske, D. W. (1959). Convergent and discriminant validation by the multitrait-multimethod matrix. *Psychol. Bull.*, **56**, 81–105.

Casement, P. (1985). Learning from the Patient. New York: Guilford Press.

Cassel, C. & Ruben, D. (2011). Specialization, subspecialization, and subsubspecialization in internal medicine. *N. Eng. J. Med.*, **364**(12), 1169–1173.

Chambless, D. & Hollon, S. (1998). Defining empirically supportable therapies. *J. Consult. Clin. Psychol.*, **66**, 7–18.

Chan, P. D., Thomas, D. M., McKinley, E. W., & Stanford, E. K., eds. (2001). Outpatient and Primary Care Medicine. Laguna Hills, CA: Current Clinical Strategies Publications.

Charon, R. (2006). Narrative Medicine: Honoring the Stories of Illness, pp. 413–421. New York: Oxford University Press.

Cheek, J. M. (1982). Aggregation, moderator variables, and the validity of personality tests: a peer-rating study. *J. Pers. Soc. Psychol.*, **43**, 1254–1269.

Cohen, J. (1988). Statistical Power for the Behavioral Sciences, 2nd edn. Hillsdale, NJ: Erlbaum.

de Jonge, P., Huyse, F. J., & Stiefel, F. C. (2006). Case and care complexity in the medically ill. *Med. Clin. North Am.*, **90**, 679–692.

Derogatis, L. R. (2000). Symptom Checklist-90-Revised. Saddle River, NJ: Pearson Education.

Donnay, D. A. C., Morris, M. L., Schaubhut, N. A., & Thompson, R. C. (2005). Strong Interest Inventory Manual: Research, Development, and Strategies for Interpretation, rev. edn. Palo Alto, CA: Consulting Psychologists Press.

Downie, S. & Mcnaughton, J. (2000). Clinical Judgement: Evidence in Practice. Oxford: Oxford University Press.

Elkin, I., Shea, M. T., Watkins, J. T., *et al.* (1989). National Institute of Mental Health Treatment of Depression Collaborative Research Program: general effectiveness of treatments. *Arch. Gen. Psychiatry*, **46**(11), 971–982.

Epstein, S. (1983). Aggregation and beyond: some basic issues on the prediction of behavior. *J. Pers.*, **51**, 360–392.

Faraone, S. V. & Tsuang, M. T. (1994). Measuring diagnostic accuracy in the absence of a "gold standard." *Am. J. Psychiatry*, **151**, 650–657.

Fauci, A., Braunwald, E., Kasper, D., *et al.*, eds. (2008). Harrison's Principles of Internal Medicine, 17th edn. New York: McGraw-Hill.

Fava, G. A., Sonino, N., & Wise, T. N. (2011). The Psychometric Assessment: Strategies to Improve Clinical Practice (Advances in Psychosomatic Medicine). Basel: Karger AG.

Folensbee, R. (2007). The Neuroscience of Psychological Therapies. Cambridge: Cambridge University Press.

Fonagy, P. (2006). Evidence-based psychodynamic psychotherapies. In PDM Task Force, eds., Psychodynamic Diagnostic Manual, pp. 765–819. Silver Spring, MD: Alliance of Psychoanalytic Organizations.

Fox, E. (2008). Emotion Science. Basingstoke: Palgrave Macmillan.

Frank, J. D. & Frank, J. B. (1991). Persuasion and Healing, 3rd edn. Baltimore, MD: Johns Hopkins University Press.

Frankel, R. (2004). Relationship-centered care and the patient-physician relationship. *J. Gen Intern. Med.*, **19**(11), 1163–1165.

Frankel, R. & Inui, T. (2006). Re-forming relationships in health care. *J. Gen. Intern. Med.*, **21 Suppl. 1**, S1–S2.

Frankel, R., Quill, T., & McDaniel, S. (2003). The Biopsychosocial Approach: Past, Present, and Future. Rochester, NY: University of Rochester Press.

Frankel, S. (1995). Intricate Engagements: The Collaborative Basis of Therapeutic Change. Northvale, NJ: Aronson.

Frankel, S. (2000). Hidden Faults: Recognizing and Resolving Therapeutic Disjunctions. Madison, CT: International Universities Press.

Frankel, S. (2007). Making Psychotherapy Work: Collaborating Successfully with Your Patient. Madison, CT: International Universities Press.

Frankel, S. (2008). Evidence from Within: A Paradigm for Clinical Practice. New York: Rowman & Littlefield.

Gabrielli, A., Avvedimento, E. V., & Krieg, T. (2009). Scleroderma. *N. Engl. J. Med.*, **360**, 1989–2003.

Garb, H. N. (1984). The incremental validity of information used in personality assessment. *Clin. Psychol. Rev.*, **4**, 641–655.

Gawande, A. (2003). Complications: A Surgeon's Notes on an Imperfect Science. New York: Picador (Macmillan).

Gawande, A. (2007, May 10). Curing the system. *The New York Times* (Opinion), www.nytimes.com/2007/05/10/opinion/19gawande.html, accessed May 18, 2012.

Gawande, A., Fisher, E. S., Gruber, J., & Rosenthal, M. B. (2009). The cost of health care: highlights from a discussion about economics and reform. *N. Engl. J. Med.*, **361**(15), 1421–1423.

Gelso, C. (2009). The real relationship in the postmodern world: theoretical and empirical explorations. *Psychother. Res.*, **19**(3), 253–264.

Gitlin, D. F., Levenson, J. L., & Lyketos, C. G. (2004). Psychosomatic medicine: a new psychiatric subspecialty. *Acad. Psychiatry*, **28**, 4–11.

Gittell, J. H. (2009). High Performance Healthcare: Using the Power of Relationships to Achieve Quality, Efficiency and Resilience. New York: McGraw Hill.

Gittell, J. H., Fairfield, K. M., Bierbaum, B., *et al.* (2000). Impact of relational coordination on quality of care, postoperative pain and functioning, and length of stay: a nine-hospital study of surgical patients. *Med. Care*, **38**(8), 807–819.

Gittell, J. H., Weinberg, D. B., Bennett, A. L., & Miller, J. A. (2008). Is the doctor in? A relational approach to job design and the coordination of work. *Hum. Resource Manage.*, **47**(4), 729–755.

Goldberg, L. R. & Werts, C. E. (1966). The reliability of clinicians' judgments: a multitrait-multimethod approach. *J. Consult. Psychol.*, **30**, 199–206.

Grant, R. W., Ashburner, J. M., Hong, C. C., *et al.* (2011). Defining patient complexity from the primary care physician's perspective: a cohort study. *Ann. Intern. Med.*, **155**, 797–804.

Grantcharov, T., Rasti, Z., Rossen, B., Kristensen, V., & Rosenberg, J. (2002). Interobserver agreement in ultrasound examination of the biliary tract. *Acta Radiol.*, **43**(1), 77–79.

Greenberg, J. (1986). The problem of analytic neutrality. *Contemp. Psychoanal.*, **22**, 76–86.

Greenberg, J. (1999). Analytic authority and analytic restraint. *Contemp. Psychoanal.*, **35**(1), 25–42.

Groopman, S. (2007, January 29). What's the trouble: how doctors think. *The New Yorker*, www.newyorker.com/reporting/2007/01/29/070129fa_fact_groopman, accessed May 18, 2012.

Grotstein, J. (1981). Splitting and Projective Identification. New York: Jason Aronson.

Hamilton, M. (1960). A rating scale for depression. *Neurol. Neurosurg. Psychiat.*, **23**, 56–62. doi: 10.1136/jmmp.23.1.56

Hashizume, H., Horibe, T., Ohshima, A., *et al.* (2005). Anxiety accelerates T-helper 2-tilted immune responses in patients with atopic dermatitis. *Br. J. Dermatol.*, **152**(6), 1161–1164.

Haug, M. R. & Lavin, B. (1979). Public challenge of physician authority. *Med. Care*, **17**(8), 844–858.

Haywood, K. L., Staniszewska, S., & Chapman, S. (2012). Quality and acceptability of patient-reported outcome measures used in chronic fatigue syndrome/myalgic encephalomyelitis (CFS/ME): a systematic review. *Qual. Life Res.*, **21**(1), 35–52.

Henderson, R. & Keiding, H. (2005). Individual survival time prediction using statistical methods. *J. Med. Ethics*, **31**, 703–706.

Herman, J. L. (1992). Trauma and Recovery. New York: Basic Books.

Hill, C. E. & Lambert, M. J. (2004). Methodological issues in studying psychotherapy processes and outcomes. In M. J. Lambert, ed., Bergin and Garfield's Handbook of Psychotherapy and Behavior Change, 5th edn., pp. 72–114. New York: John Wiley & Sons.

Hilsenroth, M. (2007). A programmatic study of short-term psychodynamic psychotherapy: assessment, process, outcome, and training. *Psychother. Res.*, **17**, 31–45.

Hilsenroth, M. & Cromer, T. (2007). Clinical interventions related to alliance during the initial interview and psychological assessment. *Psychotherapy (Chic.)*, **44**(2), 205–218.

Hinami, K., Whelan, C. T., Konetzka, R. T., *et al.* (2010). Effects of provider characteristics on care coordination under comanagement. *J. Hosp. Med.*, **5**(9), 508–513.

Hoffman, I. (1996). The intimate and ironic authority of the psychoanalyst's presence. *Psychoanal. Q.*, **65**, 102–136.

Hoffman, I. (1998). Ritual and Spontaneity in the Psychoanalytic Process: A Dialectical-Constructivist View. Hillsdale, NJ: Analytic Press.

Hummel, T. J. (1999). The usefulness of tests in clinical decisions. In J. W. Lichtenberg & R. K. Goodyear, eds., Scientist-Practitioner Perspectives on Test Interpretation, pp. 59–112. Boston, MA: Allyn & Bacon.

Hussey, P. S., Eibner, C., Ridgely, M. S., & McGlynn, E. A. (2009). Perspective: controlling U.S. health care spending – separating promising from unpromising approaches. N. Engl. J. Med., 361, 2109–2111.

Huyse, F. J., Stiefel, F. C., & de Jonge, P. (2006). Identifiers, or "red flags" of complexity and need for integrated care. Med. Clin. North Am., 90(4), 703–712.

Institute of Medicine of the National Academies (2001). Crossing the Quality Chasm: A New Health System for the 21st Century. Washington DC: National Academies Press.

Kahn, N. B. Jr. (2004). The future of family medicine: a collaborative project of the Family Medicine Community. Ann. Fam. Med., 2 Suppl. 1, S3–S32. doi: 10.1370/afm.130

Kates, N., McPherson-Doe, C., & George, L. (2011). Integrating mental health services within primary care settings: the Hamilton Family Health Team. J. Ambul. Care Manage., 34(2), 174–182.

Kathol, R. & Gatteau, S. (2007). Healing Mind and Body: A Critical Issue for Health Care Reform. Westport, CT: Praeger/Greenwood.

Kathol, R. G., Kunkel, E. J., Weiner, J. S., et al. (2009). Psychiatrists for medically complex patients: bringing value at the physical health and mental health substance use disorder interface. Psychosomatics, 50, 93–107.

Kathol R. G., Perez, R., & Cohen, J. (2010a). The Integrated Case Management Manual: Assisting Complex Patients Regain Physical and Mental Health. New York: Springer.

Kathol, R. G., Butler, M., McAlpine, D. D., & Kane, R. L. (2010b). Barriers to physical and mental condition integrated service delivery. Psychosom. Med., 72, 511.

Katon, W. & Unützer, J. (2011). Consultation psychiatry in the medical home and accountable care organizations: achieving the triple aim. Gen. Hosp. Psychiatry, 33, 305–310.

Katon, W., Von Korff, M., & Lin, E. (1990). Distressed high utilizers of medical care: DSM III diagnoses and treatment needs. Gen. Hosp. Psychiatry, 12, 355–362.

Katon, W., Robinson, P., Von Korff, M., et al. (1996). A multifaceted intervention to improve treatment of depression in primary care. Arch. Gen. Psychiatry, 53, 924–932.

Katon, W., Von Korff, M., Lin, E., et al. (1999). Stepped collaborative care for primary care patients with persistent symptoms of depression: a randomized trial. Arch. Gen. Psychiatry, 56, 1109–1115.

Katon, W., Von Korff, M., Lin, E., et al. (1995). Collaborative management to achieve treatments guidelines: the impact of depression in primary care. JAMA, 273, 1026–1031.

Kazdin, A. E. (1998). Research Design in Clinical Psychology, 3rd edn. New York: Allyn & Bacon.

Knaup, C., Koesters, M., Becker, T., & Ptschner, B. (2009). The effect of feedback of treatment outcome in specialist mental healthcare: meta-analysis. Br. J. Psychiatry, 195, 15–22.

Kovner, A. R. (2010). What more evidence do you need? Harv. Bus. Rev., 88(5), 123–127.

Kovner, A. R., Elton, J. J., & Billings, J. (2000). Evidence-based management. Front. Health Serv. Manage., 16(4), 3–24.

Krupnick, J. L., Sotsky, S. M., Simmens, S., et al. (1996). The role of the therapeutic alliance in psychotherapy and pharmacotherapy outcomes: findings in the National Institute of Mental Health treatment of depression collaborative research program. J. Consult. Clin. Psychol., 64, 532–539.

La Barre, F. (2001). On Moving and Being Moved: Nonverbal Behavior in Clinical Practice. Hillsdale, NJ: Analytic Press.

Latour, C. H., van der Windt, D. A., de Jonge, P., *et al.* (2007a). Nurse-led case management for ambulatory complex patients in general health care: a systematic review. *J. Psychosom. Res.*, **62**(3), 385–395.

Latour, C. H., Bosmans, J. E., van Tulder, M. W., *et al.* (2007b). Cost-effectiveness of a nurse-led case-management intervention in general-medical outpatients compared with usual care: an economic evaluation alongside a randomized, controlled trial. *J. Psychosom. Res.*, **62**(3), 363–370.

Lazarus, A. & Zur, O., eds. (2002). Dual Relationships and Psychotherapy. New York: Springer.

Leder, D. (1990). Clinical interpretation: the hermeneutics of medicine. *Theor. Med. Bioeth.*, **11**(1), 9–24.

Leentjens, A. F. G., Rundell, J. R., Wolcott, D. L., *et al.* (2011). Psychosomatic medicine and consultation-liaison psychiatry: scope of practice, processes, and competencies for psychiatrists or psychosomatic medicine specialists. A consensus statement of the European Association of Consultation-Liaison Psychiatry and Psychosomatics (EACLPP) and the Academy of Psychosomatic Medicine (APM). Reprint. *J. Psychosom. Res.*, **70** (5), 486–491.

Leff, B., Reider, L., Frick, K. D., *et al.* (2009). Guided care and the cost of complex healthcare: a preliminary report. *Am. J. Manag. Care*, **15**(8), 555–559.

Matthews, G., ed. (1997). Science and Emotions: Cognitive Science Perspectives on Personality and Emotion. Amsterdam: Elsevier.

May, T. (1995). The basis and limits of physician authority: a reply to critics. *J. Med. Ethics*, **21**(3), 170–173.

McGrady, A., Olson, R. P., & Kroon, J. S. (1995). Biobehavioral treatment of essential hypertension. In M. S. Schwartz, ed., Biofeedback: A Practitioner's Guide, 2nd edn., pp. 445–467. New York: Guilford Press.

McMillan, J. (2004). Educational Research: Fundamentals for the Consumer, 4th edn., pp. 227–228. Boston, MA: Allyn & Bacon.

Meyer, G. J. (2003). The reliability and validity of the Rorschach and Thematic Apperception Test (TAT) compared to other psychological and medical procedures: an analysis of systematically gathered evidence. In M. Hilsenroth & D. Segal, vol. eds., & M. Hersen series ed., Comprehensive Handbook of Psychological Assessment, vol. 2, Personality Assessment, pp. 315–342. Hoboken, NJ: JohnWiley & Sons.

Meyer, G. J., Finn, S. E., Eyde, L. D., *et al.* (2001). Psychological testing and psychological assessment: a review of evidence and issues. *Am. Psychol.*, **56**(2), 128–165.

Millon, T. (1996). Disorders of Personality: DSM IV and Beyond. New York: John Wiley & Sons.

Mitchell, S. (1997). Influence and Autonomy in Psychoanalysis. Hillsdale, NJ: Analytic Press.

Mitchell, S. (1998). The analyst's knowledge and authority. *Psychoanal. Q.*, **68**, 1–31.

Mitchell, S. A. & Aron, L. (1999). Relational Psychoanalysis: The Emergence of a Tradition. Hillsdale, NJ: Analytic Press.

Morey, L. C. (2007). The Personality Assessment Inventory Professional Manual. Lutz, FL: Psychological Assessment Resources.

Moumjid, G., Bremond, A., & Carrere, M. (2007). Seeking a second opinion: do patients need a second opinion when policy guidelines exist? *Health Policy*, **80**(1), 43–50.

Murray, H. (1943). Thematic Apperception Test. Cambridge, MA: Harvard University Press.

Myers-Briggs, I. (1962). The Myers-Briggs Type Indicator. Palo Alto, CA: Consulting Psychologists Press.

Najavits, L. M. & Strupp, H. H. (1994). Differences in the effectiveness of psychodynamic therapies: a process-outcome study. *Psychotherapy,* **31**(1), 114–123.

Naughton, B. J., Moran, M. B., Feinglass, J., Falconer, J., & Williams, M. E. (1994). Reducing hospital costs for the geriatric patient admitted from the emergency department: a randomized trial. *J. Am. Geriatr. Soc.,* **42**, 1045–1049.

Norcross, J. C., ed. (2002). Psychotherapy Relationships that Work: Therapist Contributions and Responsiveness to Patients, pp. 3–16. New York: Oxford.

Norcross, J. C., Beutler, L. E., & Levant, R. F. (2006). Evidence-based Practices in Mental Health. Washington DC: American Psychological Association.

Novotny, C. & Thompson-Brenner, H. (2004). The empirical status of empirically supported psychotherapies: assumptions, findings, and reporting in controlled clinical trials. *Psych. Bull.,* **130**, 631–663.

Nutting, P., Miller, W., Crabtree, B. F., *et al.* (2009). Initial lessons from the first national demonstration project on practice transformation to a patient-centered medical home. *Ann. Fam. Med.,* **7**(3), 254–260.

Ogden, T. (1982). Projective Identification and Psychotherapeutic Technique. Northvale, NJ: Aronson.

Olges, B. M., Lambert, M. J., & Sawyer, J. D. (1995). Clinical significance of the National Institute of Mental Health Treatment of Depression Collaborative Research Program data. *J. Consult. Clin. Psychol.,* **63**, 321–326.

Orange, D., Atwood, G., & Stolorow, R. (1997). Working Intersubjectively: Contextualism in Psychoanalytic Practice. Hillsdale, NJ: Analytic Press.

Pellerin, M.-A., Elwyn, G., Rousseau, M., *et al.* (2011). Toward shared decision making: using the OPTION scale to analyze resident-patient consultations in family medicine. *Acad. Med.,* **86**(8), 1010–1018.

Peskin, H. (2012). "Man Is a Wolf to Man": disorders of dehumanization in psychoanalysis. *Psychoanal. Dialog.,* **22**(2), 190–205.

Plsek, P. E. & Greenhalgh, T. (2001). Complexity science: the challenge of complexity in health care. *BMJ,* **323**, 625–628.

Reichenbach, D. J., Tackett, D., Harris, J., *et al.* (2006). Laparoscopic colon resection early in the learning curve: what is the appropriate setting? *Ann. Surg.,* **243**(6), 730–737.

Renik, O. (1993). Analytic interaction: conceptualizing technique in light of the analyst's irreducible subjectivity. *Psychoanal. Q.,* **62**, 553–571.

Ritter, F. E. & Schooler, L. J. (2001). The learning curve. In N. J. Smelser & P. B. Baltes, eds., International Encyclopedia of the Social and Behavioral Sciences, pp. 8602–8605. Oxford, UK: Elsevier.

Robinson, P., Wilson, D., Coral, A., Murphy, A., & Verow, P. (1999). Variation between experienced observers in the interpretation of accident and emergency radiographs. *Br. J. Radiol.,* **72**(856), 323–330.

Rogers, J. (2008). The patient-centered medical home movement: promise and peril for family medicine. *J. Am. Board Fam. Med.,* **21**(5), 370–374.

Rorschach, H. (1921). Psychodiagnostik. Bern, Switzerland: Bircher Verlag.

Roter, D. (2000). The enduring and evolving nature of the patient-physician relationship. *Patient Educ. Couns.,* **39**(1), 5–15.

Roth, A. & Fonagy, P. (2005). What Works for Whom, 2nd edn. New York: Guilford Press.

Rorty, R. (1991). Objectivity, Relativism, and Truth, vols. 1 & 2. Cambridge, UK: Cambridge University Press.

Rundell, J. R. (2010). Integrated practice model outcomes compared with traditional consultation models. *J. Psychosom. Res*, **68**, 661.

Rundell, J. R., Amundsen, K., Rummans, T. L., & Tennen, G. (2008). Toward defining the scope of psychosomatic medicine practice: psychosomatic medicine in an outpatient, tertiary-care practice setting. *Psychosomatics*, **49**, 487–493.

Safford, M. M., Allison, J. J., & Klefe, C. I. (2007). Patient complexity: more than comorbidity. The vector model of complexity. *J. Gen. Intern. Med.*, **22 Suppl. 3**, 382–390.

Shaller, D. (2007). Patient-centered care: what does it take? (On line). *Commonw. Fund*, **74**, October 24, www.commonwealthfund.org/Publications/Fund-Reports/2007/Oct/Patient-Centered-Care--What-Does-It-Take.aspx, accessed May 18, 2012.

Stange, K. C., Nutting, P. A., Miller, W. L., *et al.* (2010). Defining and measuring the patient-centered medical home. *J. Gen. Intern. Med.*, **25**(6), 601–612.

Stiefel, F. C., Huyse, F. J., Sollner, W., *et al.* (2006). Operationalizing integrated care on a clinical level: the INTERMED Project. *Med. Clin. North Am.*, **90**(4), 713–758.

Stolorow, R. D., Atwood, G. E., & Orange, D. M. (2002). Worlds of Experience: Interweaving Philosophical and Clinical Dimensions in Psychoanalysis. New York: Basic Books.

Straus, S. E., Glasziou, M. B., Richardson, W. S., & Haynes, R. B. (2010). Evidence-based Medicine: How to Practice and Teach It, 4th edn. Philadelphia, PA: Churchill Livingstone Elsevier.

Strenger, C. (1991). Between Hermeneutics and Science: An Essay on the Epistemology of Psychoanalysis. New York: International Universities Press.

Sturm, R., Unützer, J., & Katon, W. (1999). Effectiveness research and implications for study design: sample size and statistical power. *Gen. Hosp. Psychiatry*, **21**, 274–283.

Sullivan, M. (2003). The new subjective medicine: taking the patient's point of view in health care. *Soc. Sci. Med.*, **56**(7), 1595–1604.

Tanenbaum, S. J. (1993). What physicians know. *N. Engl. J. Med.*, **329**, 1268–1271.

van der Kolk, B. (1988). The trauma spectrum: the interaction of biological and social events in the genesis of the trauma response. *J. Trauma. Stress*, **1**(3), 273–290.

van der Kolk, B. (2002). Posttraumatic therapy in the age of neuroscience. *Psychoanal. Dialog.*, **12**, 381–392.

Verghese, A. (2002, December 8). The healing paradox: The way we live now. *The New York Times Magazine*, www.nytimes.com/2002/12/08/magazine/08WWLN.html, accessed May 18, 2012.

Vogeli, C., Shields, A. E., & Lee, T. A. (2007). Multiple chronic conditions: prevalence, health consequences, and implications for quality, care management, and costs. *J. Gen. Intern. Med.*, **22 Suppl. 3**, 391–395.

Wampold, B. E. (2001). The Great Psychotherapy Debate: Models, Methods, and Findings. Mahwah, NJ: Erlbaum.

Watson, J. & Rennie, D. (1994). Quantitative analysis of clients' subjective experience of significant moments during the exploration of problematic reactions. *J. Counseling Psych.*, **41**, 500–509.

Wechsler, D. (1987). Wechsler Memory Scale – Revised. San Antonio, TX: The Psychological Corp.

Weinberger, J. & Westen, D. (2004). When clinical description becomes statistical prediction. *Am. Psychol.*, **59**, 595–613.

Westen, D. & Bradley, R. (2005). Empirically supported complexity: rethinking evidence-based psychotherapy. *Curr. Dir. Psychol. Sci.*, **14**, 266–271.

Westen, D., Heim, A. K., Morrison, K., Patterson, M., & Campbell, L. (2002). Simplifying diagnosis using a prototype-matching approach: implications for the next edition of the DSM. In L. E. Beutleler & M. L. Malik, eds., Rethinking the DSM: A Psychological Perspective, pp. 221–250. Washington DC: American Psychological Association.

White, S. & Stancombe, J. (2003). Clinical Judgement in the Health and Welfare Professions: Extending the Evidence Base. Maidenhead, UK: Open University Press.

Winblad, U. (2008). Do physicians care about patient choice? *Soc. Sci. Med.*, **67**(10), 1502–1511.

Woolf, S. H. & George, J. N. (2000). Evidence-based medicine: interpreting studies and setting policy. *Hematol. Oncol. Clin. North Am.*, **14**(4), 761–784.

Wulsin, L. R., Söllner, W., & Pincus, H. A. (2006). Models of integrated care: review. *Med. Clin. North Am.*, **90**(4), 647–677.

Zatzick, D., Roy-Byrne, P., Russo, J., *et al.* (2004). A randomized effectiveness trial of stepped collaborative care for acutely injured trauma survivors. *Arch. Gen. Psychiatry*, **61**, 498–506.

Zatzick, D., Rivara, F., Jurkovich, G., *et al.* (2011). Enhancing the population impact of collaborative care interventions: mixed method development and implementation of stepped care targeting posttraumatic stress disorder and related comorbidities after acute trauma. *Gen. Hosp. Psychiatry*, **33**, 123–134.

Zeber, J. E., Miller, A. L., Copeland, L. A., *et al.* (2011). Medication adherence, ethnicity, and the influence of multiple psychosocial and financial barriers. *Admin. Pol. Ment. Health*, **38**(2), 86–95.

Zur, O. (2011). Dual Relationships, Multiple Relationships and Boundaries in Psychotherapy, Counseling and Mental Health. Sonoma, CA: Zur Institute. Retrieved March 24, 2011 from www.zurinstitute.com/dualrelationships.html.

Index

accountability of the physician 7
  truing required
    by patients 129–30
addiction *see* case studies, Mary
adjustment disorder *see* case studies, Neal
affordability of MPCP care 161–2
agendas, influence on clinical
    interactions 69
algorithms to guide treatment 25, 36–7
  limitations in clinical practice 51
  limitations in complex cases 63
  manualized protocols 49–50
American Academy of Family Physicians 4
American Diabetes Association 5–6
anxiety *see* case studies, Lucy; case studies,
  Nathan
asymptote concept 13
attention deficit disorder *see* case studies, Victor
attention deficit/hyperactivity disorder (ADHD)
  see case studies, Larry; case studies, Neal

Beck Depression Inventory-II (BSI-II) 42
best practice guidelines 25
bipolar disorder 10–12
  see also case studies, Stanley; case studies,
  Victor

care delivery
  appropriate cases for MPCP care 150–3
  comprehensive treatment protocol 145–7
  implementation of the MPCP model 167–8
  influence of the MPCP 134–9
  models of care 3–4
  MPCP model 3–4
  MPCP role in complex cases 148
case studies
  Alan 51–4, 59, 63–4, 69, 71–2, 75, 81, 85,
    110–11, 131
  Alison 106–7, 109, 111–12
  Diane 38

Dorothy 38–9, 127–8
examples of appropriate MPCP cases 150–3
Flora 39–40
Hilary 141–3
John 51
Joshua 40–1
Keith 27–32, 34, 85–6, 88–9, 92, 108–9, 127, 130
Larry 134–9, 143–4
Lucy 75–6
Margie 45–7
Marty 111–12, 116, 129–30
Mary 44–5, 47
Michael 119–22
Natalie 112–17, 122, 127
Nathan 107–8, 123–5, 127, 130, 134–9,
  143, 146–7
Neal 54–64, 70–2, 77–9, 83–4, 87–9,
  98–102, 126, 139–40
Nel 30–4
Randy 22–3
Solomon 65–6, 72, 77, 83–5, 91–2, 94–8,
  102–6, 110, 139–40
Stanley 9–10, 14–16, 151–3
Victor 42–3
childhood sexual abuse *see* case studies, Natalie
chronic fatigue syndrome *see* case studies, Joshua
clinical accuracy
  contribution of truing devices 127–9, 142
  use of truing measures 139–40
clinical assessment, false positives and false
  negatives 38–41
clinical complexity 1–3, 148
  and clinical judgment 76
  and the MPCP role 133
  and treatment strategy 66–8
  dimensions of 19–23
  sources of 19–20
  use of the SO framework 76–9
  see also case studies, Alan; case studies,
  Neal; case studies, Solomon

clinical decision making 49–51, 76
    clinical judgment 8
    incremental validity 48
    practical dilemma for physicians 82
    see also treatment decisions
clinical experience, and the MPCP role 79–80
clinical intuition
    and experience-based clinical judgment
        (EBCJ) 78
    and physician choices 79–80
    versus strategy 71–2
clinical judgment 49
    and clinical complexity 76
    and clinical strategy 9–13, 90
    and intuition 78–80
    and physician choices 79–80
    and the MPCP role 85–6
    effects of failure 85–6
    interaction with truing measures 130–1
    linking with truing measures 123–6
    objective and subjective components 8
    role of clinical judgment 85
    selection of truing mechanisms 88–9
    successful case 87–8
    support from truing measures 79–80, 84–5
clinical measurement, successive approximations
        13
clinical practice
    contributions from the patient 73
    contributions from the physician 73
    factors affecting precision 130–1
    influence of subjectivity 74
    inherent complexity 65
    limitations of algorithms 51
    list of factors at play 72–4
    non-verbal aspects 73
    outcome measures 89
    person-specific variables 14–16
    realities of 146–7
    role of subjectivity 14–16
    use of algorithms (manualized protocols)
        49–50
clinical progress
    and the conjunctive sequence 126–7
    continuities and discontinuities 126–7
    interpersonal experiences 126–7
    monitoring 143–5
clinical standards 16–17
clinical strategy
    and clinical complexity 66–8
    and clinical intuition 71–2
    and clinical judgment 9–13, 90

and interpersonal collaboration 70–1
and the physician–patient relationship
        91–102
complex interpersonal aspects 91–3
definitions 91
emerging complications 93–4
in psychiatry (Neal) 98–102
leadership role 70–1
MPCP perspective 91–3, 102–4
primary care interface with psychiatry
        (Solomon) 94–8
subjective complications 93–4
support from truing methods 102
clinical testing
    ambiguity in 37–8
    as a truing device 47
    truing methods 37
clinical tools, range of tools available 48–9
clinical truth, and truing devices 13
CNS-based illness and psychiatry 5
cognitive behavioral therapy (CBT) 50–1, 55
collaborative care xi–xii
    and the MPCP 63–4
    coordination by the MPCP 102–4, 156–7
    Level 2 truing by the MPCP 140–1
    see also physician–patient collaboration;
        treatment team
communication, role of the MPCP 53–4, 85
co-morbid systemic medical and psychiatric
        illnesses 1–2
complex cases
    and the MPCP model of care 3–4, 148
    definition 17–18
    examples of appropriate MPCP cases 150–3
    limitations of evidence-based treatment
        protocols 63
    models of care 3–4
    need for the MPCP 1–2
    steps in evolution of 54–64
    truing sequence in a complex case 54–64
    utilization of healthcare resources 1–2
complex partial seizures *see* case studies, Larry
complex patients, definition 148
complexity
    dimensions in clinical work 2–3
    see also clinical complexity; diagnostic
        complexity; management complexity;
        operational complexity
comprehensive personality and
    neuropsychological assessment
    components of 42
    unlocking complex cases 42–7

comprehensive treatment protocol, and the
  MPCP 145–6
conjunctive sequence
  and clinical progress 126–7
  at MPCP level 135
  physician–patient alliance 120–2
consensus *see* physician–patient consensus
continuous quality improvement 26
coordinating physician model 4, 133, 149, 155
costs, impact of MPCP management 161–2
countertransferences, influence on clinical
  interactions 69
cyclothymic disorder *see* case studies, Stanley

decision making *see* clinical decision making;
  treatment decisions
decision trees 25*see also* algorithms
delivery of care *see* care delivery
dependent variable in medicine 7–8
depression *see* case studies, Mary; case studies,
  Neal; case studies, Victor
depressive disorder *see* case studies, Larry
diabetes mellitus
  diagnostic criteria 5–6
  integrated approach to treatment 6–8
  see also case studies, Michael
diagnosis and treatment
  approaches to 29–30
  patient's perspective on 127–9
diagnostic ambiguity *see* case studies, Alison
*Diagnostic and Statistical Manual of Mental
  Disorders* (DSM-IV-TR) 49
  schizoaffective disorder 50–1
  schizophrenia 6
diagnostic complexity 2–3, 38–41
diagnostic testing *see* clinical testing
difficult-to-manage patients 17–18
dual-trained psychiatrists, appeal of the MPCP
  role 3–4

eating disorders *see* case studies, Randy
empirically-supported treatments (ESTs)
  36–7, 49–51
  limitations 81, 84–5
enactments, influence on clinical interactions 69
Erdberg, Philip 58
evidence-based guidelines 25
evidence-based medicine (EBM) 36–7
evidence-based treatments (EBTs) 36–7, 49–51
  limitations 81, 84–5, 63
executive function derangement *see* case
  studies, Larry

experience-based clinical judgment (EBCJ)
  36–7, 49, 82, 88
  and intuition 78

false negatives in clinical assessment 38–41
false positives in clinical assessment 38–41
family issues *see* case studies, Larry; case studies,
  Nathan

gambling addiction *see* case studies, Larry

Hamilton Rating Scale for Depression 42
healthcare resources, utilization by complex
  cases 1–2

imatinib 51
implementation of the MPCP model 167–8
incremental validity of clinical decisions 48
independent variables
  accounting for 7–8
  influence on clinical judgment 8
individual healthcare professional functions
  (Level 1) 2
inherent complexity 19–20
innovation and the MPCP 134
integrated treatment model of care 1–2
interferon 51
International Classification of Diseases
  (ICD-10) (WHO) 49
  schizoaffective disorder 50
inter-subjectivity between physician and
  patient 68
intuition *see* clinical intuition

laboratory testing *see* clinical testing
leadership in the clinical situation 70–1
Level 1 (microscopic) functions of the MPCP 2
Level 2 (treatment team/macroscopic) functions
  of the MPCP 2, 26–9, 130–1, 140–1, 145–6

management challenge *see* case studies, Alan
management complexity 2–3, 148
management-intensive, complex patients
  3, 17–18
medical model 29–30
medical–psychiatric coordinating physician
  (MPCP)
  affordability 161–2
  and patient-centered treatment 71
  application of the conjunctive sequence 135
  as a medical subspecialization 145, 148–9,
    158–9

becoming an MPCP 157–8
benefits in complex cases 3–4, 146–8
career paths 148–9
clinical experience required 79–80
clinical judgment 85, 138–9
clinical needs targeted 148
communication role 85
complexities of clinical work 133
complexities of the role 33–4
comprehensive treatment protocol 145–6
conflict management within the treatment team 156–7
contribution to the treatment process 34–5
coordination of care delivery 17–18
coordination of clinical strategy 91–3
coordination of complex cases 63–4
coordination of the multidisciplinary treatment team 148, 156–7
desirability of psychiatric training 153–4
evidence for need for 1–2
examples of appropriate cases 148, 150–3
features of the MPCP model of care 148
functioning of the treatment team 85–6
future development of the MPCP model 168
implementation of the MPCP model 167–8
in outpatient psychosomatic medicine 160–1
influence of patient collaboration 84
influence on the direction of treatment 134–8
innovation 134
integration of psychiatry and systemic medicine 4–5
involvement in ongoing patient care 153–4
job description 153–4
knowledge required 32
leadership role 34–5
Level 1 (microscopic) functions 2
Level 2 (treatment team/macroscopic) responsibilities 2, 26–9, 130–1, 140–1, 145–6
limits of certainty 141–3
medical training required 32
modification of the treatment plan 134–9
need for a communication facilitator 53–4
need for formalization of the role 85–6
perspective on clinical strategy 102–4
pilot study of MPCP outpatient cases 162–7
psychiatrist in the role of 3–4, 133
realities of clinical work 146–7
response to crisis situations 134–8
responsibilities 2
role in complex cases 23
role in operationally complex cases 91–3

skills required 32, 148–9, 154–6
specific training for the role 142–3
strategic role 102–4
target clinical subpopulation 3–4
therapeutic impact 134
training and experience required 153–6
training models 157–8
treatment coordinator 130–1
treatment monitoring role 79
truing at Level 2 (treatment team) 26–9, 140–1
use of outcome measures 89
use of SO analysis 78–9
medical specializations 158–9
mental dysfunctions, scope of psychiatry 5
mind-body divide, fallacy of 4–5
Minnesota Multiphasic Personality Inventory (MMPI) 42, 45–6, 124
models of care for complex cases 3–4
monitoring progress 143–5
MPCP see medical–psychiatric coordinating physician
multidisciplinary treatment team see treatment team
multiple sclerosis see case studies, Diane
myelodysplasia see case studies, Alan
myelofibrosis see case studies, Alan
Myers-Briggs Type Indicator Career Report 46

neuropsychological assessment 42, 88–9
non-verbal aspects of the clinical process 73
non-verbal contributions to consensus 116–17

one-subject scientific project see single subject research model
operational complexity 2–3, 20, 38–41, 148
organ transplantation 153
outcome criteria 89
    collaboratively defining 123–6
    measuring results 143–5
outpatient psychosomatic medicine, potential for MPCP practice 160–1

pain management see case studies, Stanley
Parkinson's disease see case studies, Nathan
patient care
    integrated treatment model (MPCP) 1–2
    place for the MPCP 1–2
    principles of 7
Patient-Centered Medical Home (PCMH) model 167–8
patient-centered treatment 36–7, 70–1

patient–physician relationship
   see physician–patient relationship
patients
  accountability of physicians 129–30
  clinical subpopulation targeted by MPCP care
   3–4
  contributions to the clinical process 73
  personal input about treatment 107–9
  reporting of their medical condition 127–9
  response to diagnosis 127–9
  suitability for MPCP care 148
personality assessment 42
Personality Assessment Inventory (PAI) 45, 124
personality disorder *see* case studies, Neal
physician
  accountability 7
  contributions to the clinical process 73
  decision-making dilemma 82
  limits of certainty 141–3
  personal accountability to patients 129–30
  role of intuition in clinical work 71–2
  subjectivity 14–16
physician–patient alliance, conjunctive sequence
  120–2
physician–patient collaboration 88–9
  as a truing device 82, 119–20
  consequences of not collaborating 107–9
  defining outcome measures 123–6
  impact on physician judgment 82–4
  patient's input about treatment 107–9
  see also case studies, Keith; case studies,
   Nathan
physician–patient consensus
  components of 117–18
  cooperation between team members 110–11
  how it works 109–12
  mixed systemic medical–psychiatric case
   112–17
  non-verbal contributions 116–17
  physician's distortions 111–12
  rapport in treatment 109
  role of truing 107
  truing measures 118
  working consensus 117–18
physician–patient reciprocity 70–1, 82–4
physician–patient relationship
  agendas 69
  and the clinical strategy 91–102
  contaminating factors 69
  countertransferences 69
  developmental stages 120–2
  dyadic versus team-based treatment 26–9

effects of uncertainty and subjectivity 64
enactments 69
interpersonal collaboration 68, 70–1
inter-subjectivity 68
leadership role 70–1
responsibility for results 70–1
responsibility for treatment 68
shared influence and responsibility 70–1
transferences 69
treatment alliance approach 67–8
physician self-discipline, Self-Other Rapid
  Assessment Method 73–5
physician self-monitoring 59, 79–80
pilot study of MPCP outpatient cases 162–7
polycythemia vera *see* case studies, Keith
posttraumatic stress disorder (PTSD) 115–16
precision in clinical work
  ambiguity in clinical testing 37–8
  and choice of truing device 139–40
  incremental validity of clinical decisions 48
  interpersonal precision 119–27, 129–31
  limits of certainty 141–3
  practical dilemma for physicians 82
  range of truing devices 13–14
  technical precision 127–31
primary care
  and systemic illnesses 5
  definition 5
  interface with psychiatry 94–8
  interpersonal factors 127
primary care physician (PCP)
  examples of complex cases 150–3
  relevance of the MPCP model 4
projective identification mechanism 73
projective testing 58
psychiatric co-morbidity, and the MPCP
  role 133
psychiatrically co-morbid, management-
  intensive, complex patients 3, 17–18,
  133
psychiatrist in the MPCP role 3–4
psychiatry
  and CNS-based illnesses 5
  and mental dysfunctions 5
  integration with systemic medicine 4–8
  interface with primary care 94–8
psychological assessment 42
  as a truing device 47
  components of 42
  factors influencing use of 49
  unlocking complex cases 42–7
psychometric testing *see* clinical testing

psychosomatic medicine, potential for MPCP practice 160–1
psychosomatic psychiatrists as MPCPs 3–4

randomized controlled trials 25
reciprocity between physician and patient 70–1, 82–4
risk-taking behavior *see* case studies, Michael
Rorschach inkblot test 42, 45–6, 124

schizoaffective disorder
    formal diagnostic criteria 50
    see also case studies, John
schizophrenia
    diagnostic criteria 6
    integrated approach to treatment 6–8
scientific approach to treatment 7–8
SCL-90 (Symptom Check List-90) 42
scleroderma *see* case studies, Solomon
Self-Other Rapid Assessment Analysis (SO Analysis) 59
    use by the MPCP 78–9
Self-Other Rapid Assessment Framework (SO framework) 73–5
    use in clinically complex contexts 76–9
Self-Other Rapid Assessment Method (SO Method) 59, 74–5, 82, 88–9
    application to systemic medicine 75–6
Self-Other Relational Configuration (SO configuration) 74–5
self-supervision method (Casement) 76
sexual abuse in childhood *see* case studies, Natalie
single-subject research model 7–8, 144
Sjögren's syndrome *see* case studies, Natalie
SO analysis *see* Self-Other Rapid Assessment Analysis
SO configuration *see* Self-Other Relational Configuration
SO framework *see* Self-Other Rapid Assessment Framework
SO method *see* Self-Other Rapid Assessment Method
Stevens–Johnson syndrome 51
strategy *see* clinical strategy
Strong Interest Inventory 46
study of MPCP outpatient cases 162–7
subjectivity in clinical work 14–16
    complicating the clinical strategy 93–4
    in the physician–patient relationship 64
    influence on the clinical process 74
    role in treatment decisions 82

substance abuse *see* case studies, Randy
systemic illness and primary care 5
systemic medicine, integration with psychiatry 4–8

technical complexity 20
Thematic Apperception Test (TAT) 42, 46
transferences, influence on clinical interactions 69
treatment algorithms *see* algorithms to guide treatment
treatment alliance 67–8, 109
    and clinical strategy 91–3
    deconstruction of the situation 109–12
    mixed systemic medical–psychiatric case 112–16
treatment approach
    integration of systemic medicine with psychiatry 6–8
    scientific argument 7–8
treatment decisions
    impact of physician–patient collaboration 82–4
    limitations of objective approaches 81
    practical dilemma in complex cases 82
    role of subjectivity 82
    use of truing devices 82
    see also clinical decision making
treatment monitoring responsibility 143–5
treatment plan
    influence of the MPCP 134–8
    modification by the MPCP 138–9
treatment strategy *see* clinical strategy
treatment team
    complexities of 27–9
    conflict management by the MPCP 156–7
    cooperation between team members 110–11
    coordination by the MPCP 17, 145–6, 148, 156–7
    Level 2 functions of the MPCP 2, 26–9, 130–1, 140–1, 145–6
    operational complexity 2–3
    truing measures 26–9, 118, 140–1
truing, definition 13
truing devices/methods/measures 1–2, 48
    and clinical truth 13
    clinical testing 37, 47
    conjunctive sequence 120–2
    consequences of omission 30–2
    contribution to clinical accuracy 88–9, 127–9, 139–40, 142

truing devices/methods/measures (cont.)
  contribution to physician–patient
    consensus 107
  definition 25–6
  factors influencing choice of 49
  incremental validity 88–9
  Level 1 (direct service providers) 26–9
  Level 2 (treatment team) 26–9, 118, 140–1
  linking with clinical judgment 79–80, 123–6,
    130–1
  list of devices 13–14
  patients' need for 129–30
  physician self-monitoring 59
  principle of successive approximations
    25–6, 48
  psychometric assessment 47, 49
  range of methods 119–20
  selection of 88–9
  support for clinical judgment 84–5, 88–9
  support for clinical strategy 102
  treatment team level 26–9, 118, 140–1
  use in treatment decision making 82
truing sequence in a complex case (Neal) 54–64
  appreciation of patient's assets 58, 63
  approach to treatment plan formulation 58–9
  descriptive distillation of patient's status
    59–60
  diagnosis 60–1
  early impressions and clinical strategy 57
  history of present illness 56
  initial contact and review of records 56
  initial impression of the patient 55
  initial intervention and treatment
    planning 57
  initial interview and clinical evaluation 56
  limitations of evidence-based treatment
    protocols 63
  medication 57
  neurological workup 57
  neuropsychological assessment 57
  physician decisions and actions 61–2
  physician self-monitoring 59
  psychometric assessments 56–8
  role of the MPCP 63–4

Wechsler Adult Intelligence Scale (WAIS-III)
  46, 124
working consensus 117–18